PREVENTING CANCER

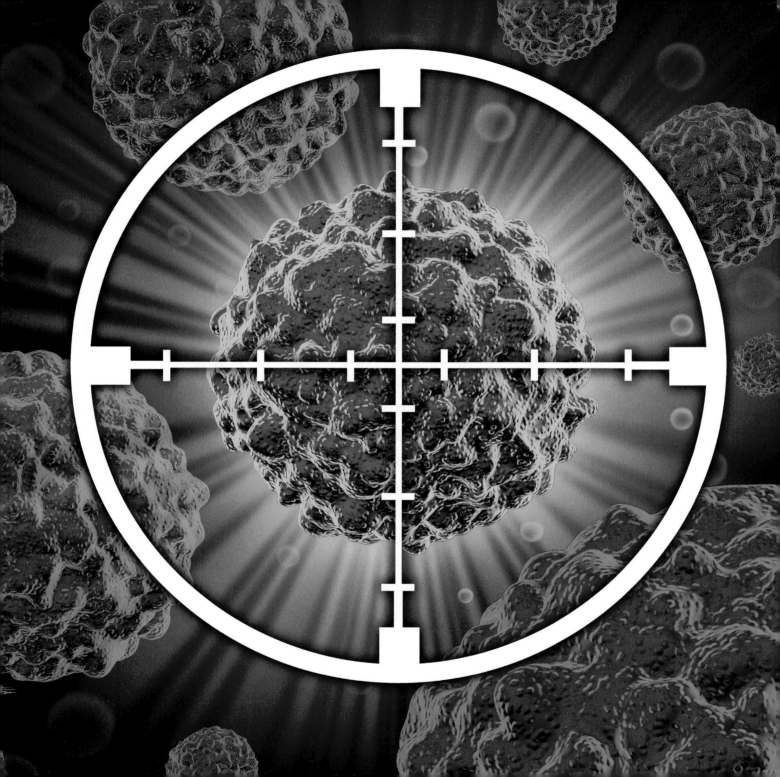

Richard Beliveau & Denis Gingras

PREVENTING CANCER
Reducing the Risks

FIREFLY BOOKS

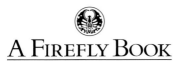

A FIREFLY BOOK

Published by Firefly Books Ltd. 2015

First printing

Publisher Cataloging-in-Publication Data (U.S.)

Béliveau, Richard, 1953-
    Preventing cancer / Richard Beliveau & Denis Gingras.
[175] pages : cm.
Includes bibliographical references.
Summary: "This guidebook explores rumors and facts surrounding cancer, what causes it and how best to treat it" – Provided by publisher.
ISBN-13: 978-1-77085-633-2 (pbk.)
1. Cancer – Prevention. I. Gingras, Denis. II. Title
616.99/405 dc23 RC268.B4413 2015

Library and Archives Canada Cataloguing in Publication

Béliveau, Richard, 1953-
[Prévenir le cancer. English]
    Preventing cancer / Richard Beliveau & Denis Gingras.
Translation of: Prévenir le cancer / Richard Béliveau Ph.D.,
    Denis Gingras Ph.D. -- Montréal (Québec): Trécarré, [2014]
Includes bibliographical references.
ISBN 978-1-77085-633-2 (paperback)
    1. Cancer--Prevention. I. Gingras, Denis, 1965-, author II. Title. II.
Title: Prévenir le cancer. English.
RC268.B4413 2015   616.99'405   C2015-902941-4

Published in the United States by
Firefly Books (U.S.) Inc.
P.O. Box 1338, Ellicott Station
Buffalo, New York 14205

Published in Canada by
Firefly Books Ltd.
50 Staples Avenue, Unit 1
Richmond Hill, Ontario L4B 0A7

Printed in Canada

Conceived, designed, and produced by
Les Éditions du Trécarré
Groupe Librex inc.
A division of Québecor Média
La Tourelle
1055, boul. René-Lévesque Est, Bureau 300
Montréal (Québec) H2L 4S5

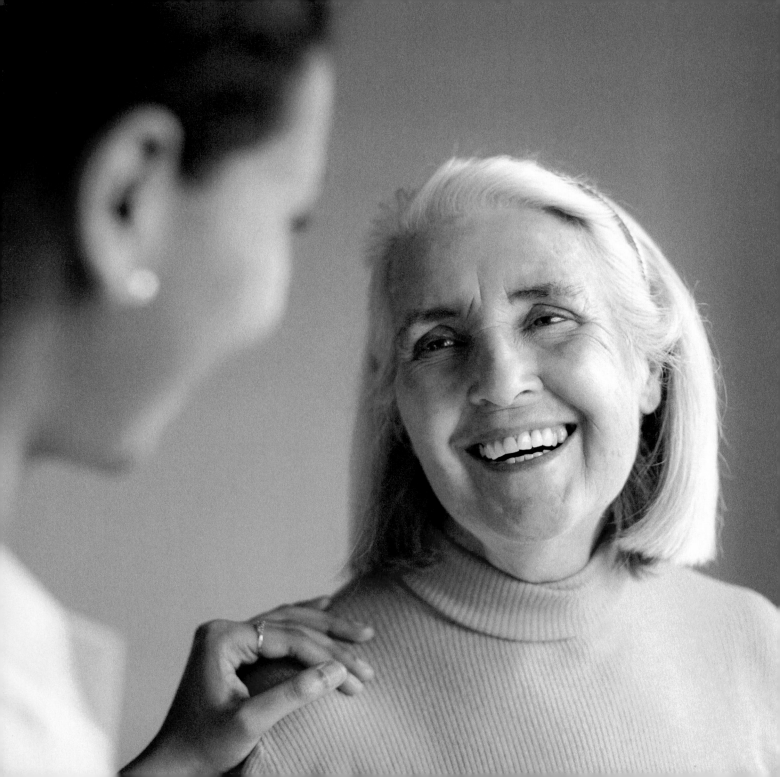

Preface

The leading cause of death in the majority of industrialized countries, cancer is one of the most difficult ordeals that many of us will have to face at some point in our lifetime. Not only does cancer threaten our very existence, it also takes away people who are dear to us, depriving us of precious moments spent in the company of family, friends and colleagues who held an important place in our lives. Cancer is truly the "grim reaper" of the 21st century, a mysterious and frightening disease whose destructive potential drains our energy and too often leaves us feeling unable to cope, resigned to its being the brutal, seemingly inevitable, end of life.

Yet there is no need for this feeling of powerlessness: thanks to what is undoubtedly one of the most important discoveries in medical research in recent years, we now know that most cancers are neither a cruel twist of fate nor an unavoidable consequence of aging, but are instead the result of the immense influence of our lifestyle on the likelihood of getting the disease. During the last 10 years, an avalanche of basic and population studies have shown beyond any doubt that the high incidence of several cancers in industrialized countries is closely related to the modern western lifestyle. The emergence and progression of cancer cells are a direct consequence of the major impacts of smoking, excess body weight, sedentary behaviors and diet. The discovery that cancer is so obviously dependent on lifestyle is a major breakthrough in the fight against the disease, as it suggest that nearly three-quarters of cancer cases currently occurring in the population could be prevented simply by changing our everyday habits, a positive impact unlikely ever to be equaled by any treatment, given the complexity of a clinically diagnosed cancer.

Despite its enormous potential, cancer prevention remains the most neglected aspect of efforts devoted to this disease. The society in which we live, focused on consumption, comfort and short-term benefits, is in some ways incompatible with a preventive approach and may even encourage lifestyle habits that run completely counter to the maintenance of good health. In most cases, therefore, prevention is a personal choice, a decision individuals make to become aware of the causes of cancer and to change their habits, so as to reduce the chance of getting the disease.

The objective of this book is to provide the necessary tools to those who want to take their fate into their own hands. Owing to the outstanding work of public health agencies like the World Cancer Research Fund and the American Cancer Society, available knowledge on cancer prevention can now be summarized in the form of 10 major recommendations with respect to smoking, body weight, physical exercise, diet and sun exposure. These recommendations, based on the rigorous analysis of several decades of cancer research, are the best weapon at our disposal to reduce dramatically the burden of cancer in our society, and for the first time give survivors of the disease a practical recurrence prevention tool to increase their life expectancy.

Cancer is a daunting enemy, and only by using all available resources, for both prevention and cure, will we really be able to make progress in the fight against this disease and reduce the pain and suffering it leaves in its wake.

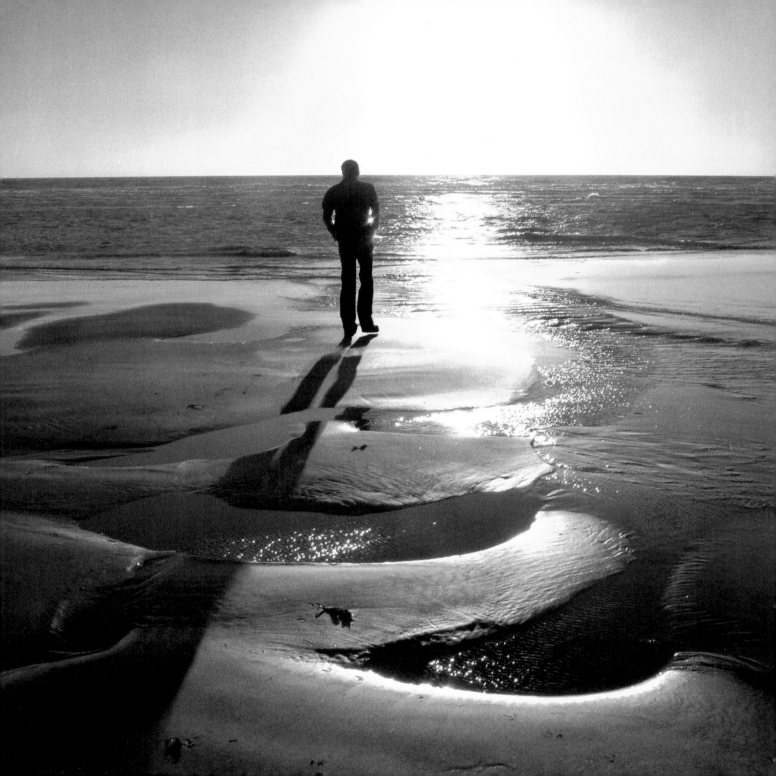

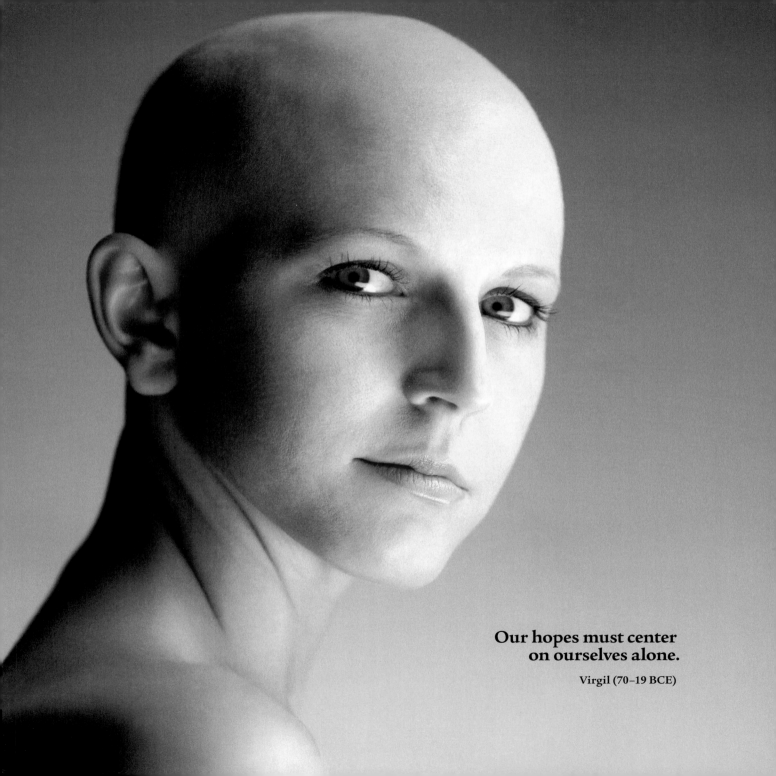

Our hopes must center
on ourselves alone.

Virgil (70–19 BCE)

Chapter 1

An Ounce of Prevention is Worth a Pound of Cure

In the tragedies of ancient Greece, characters are confronted by a series of terrible events they are powerless to change, almost as though their life stories were written in advance and it was impossible for them to escape the fate that had befallen them. More than two and a half millennia later, this concept of unavoidable destiny still influences our attitude to illness. Heart disease, diabetes and cancer, which alone cause two-thirds of all deaths in industrialized countries, are very often viewed as a cruel twist of fate or the consequences of factors outside of our control. This fatalistic view of illness has actually been reinforced in modern times by recent developments in genomics, the science that studies human genetic material. Almost every day, new genes that predispose us to particular illnesses are discovered, which can give the impression that we are programmed from birth for the health problems we experience in adulthood. Being in good health thus becomes a matter of luck, reserved for winners of the genetic lottery, while a person who is ill is always a victim of bad luck.

Attributing the events of life to pure chance or genetic predetermination is not only demoralizing, but also incorrect. With very rare exceptions — pediatric cancers or certain serious genetic diseases, for example — no aspect of

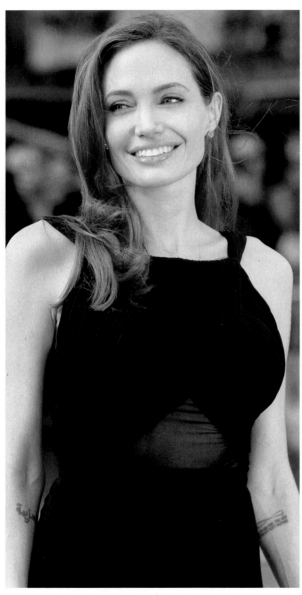

Actor, director and goodwill ambassador Angelina Jolie, a carrier of the BRCA1 gene mutation.

human life, whether it be our predispositions, our tastes or our aptitudes, is completely innate. Extraordinary progress in research in recent years shows beyond any doubt that we can be born with a gene that predisposes us to obesity or to developing cancer, but that these genes are only one of the factors involved in the onset of these diseases. The predisposition is thus very real, but it remains strongly influenced by a wide array of external factors. A striking illustration of this is the BCR-ABL oncogene, known to be the main gene responsible for chronic myeloid leukemia. Although this type of leukemia is a rare disease occurring in only a tiny portion of the population, the gene can nonetheless be detected in a third of healthy adults. The vast majority of these people never get the disease. Neither the most exhilarating nor the most difficult events of a life are written in advance; it's really our life choices that, by influencing the interaction of our genes with the external environment, are mainly responsible for the risk of getting a serious chronic disease.

Cancer, Public Enemy No. 1

Cancer is perhaps the best example of a disease whose origins are often attributed to external factors beyond our control, but which is, in most cases, the consequence of our lifestyle habits. We usually take a fatalistic approach to cancer, a reaction that is partly explained by the heavy burden it imposes. In Canada, for example, as in a number of industrialized societies, cancer has displaced heart disease as the main cause of mortality and is now responsible for roughly a third of all deaths each year, mainly because of the ravages associated with lung cancer caused by smoking, as well as colon, breast, prostate and white blood cell cancers (lymphomas) (Figure 1).

Cancer's high mortality rate reflects the difficulty in effectively treating this disease, especially when it's diagnosed at an advanced stage. This is because once it reaches this stage, a cancer consists of completely degenerated cells, which have transformed their metabolism from top to bottom to support their infinite growth and in which the chromosomes have been thrown into total anarchy, in terms of both number and integrity (Figure 2). These cells also show extensive genetic damage, with several dozen — sometimes even more than 100 — different genes modified, which makes them very hard to neutralize. Recent advances in cancer treatment have led to a slight decrease in mortality from the disease, but fighting cells that have degenerated to such a degree remains an extremely difficult task, with still uncertain results. Although we must continue to invest in research to identify new therapeutic agents, we nonetheless have to be realistic and recognize

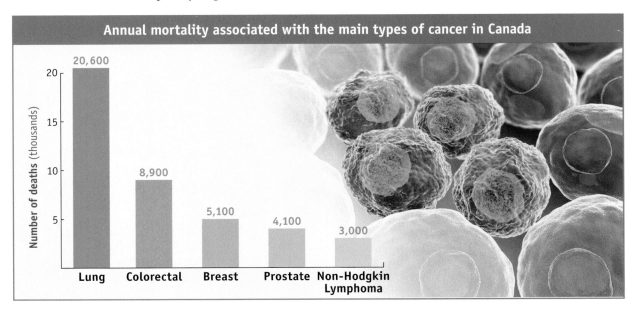

Annual mortality associated with the main types of cancer in Canada

Number of deaths (thousands)

Lung — 20,600
Colorectal — 8,900
Breast — 5,100
Prostate — 4,100
Non-Hodgkin Lymphoma — 3,000

Figure 1

that this curative approach to cancer has its limits; it's unlikely that this approach alone will ever result in a significant decrease in mortality from cancer. As with infectious diseases and heart disease before it, it is only through prevention that we will succeed in making real progress in the fight against cancer.

Stowaways

Adopting a preventive approach to cancer is all the more important given that human beings are one of the animal species most at risk of getting this disease. For example, although cancer occurs in only 2% of the great apes, one-third of the world's population will develop cancer, with this proportion even higher in some industrialized countries like Canada, where it affects 46% of men and 41%

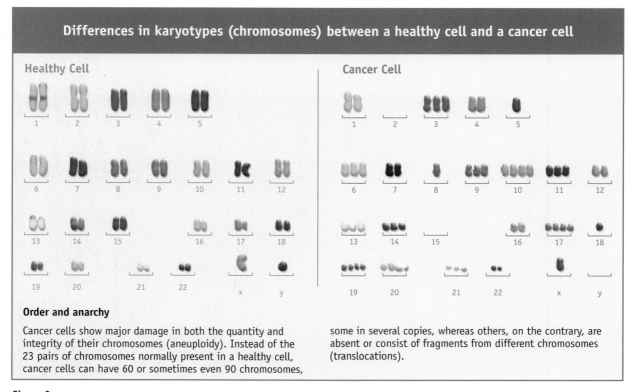

Differences in karyotypes (chromosomes) between a healthy cell and a cancer cell

Order and anarchy

Cancer cells show major damage in both the quantity and integrity of their chromosomes (aneuploidy). Instead of the 23 pairs of chromosomes normally present in a healthy cell, cancer cells can have 60 or sometimes even 90 chromosomes, some in several copies, whereas others, on the contrary, are absent or consist of fragments from different chromosomes (translocations).

Figure 2

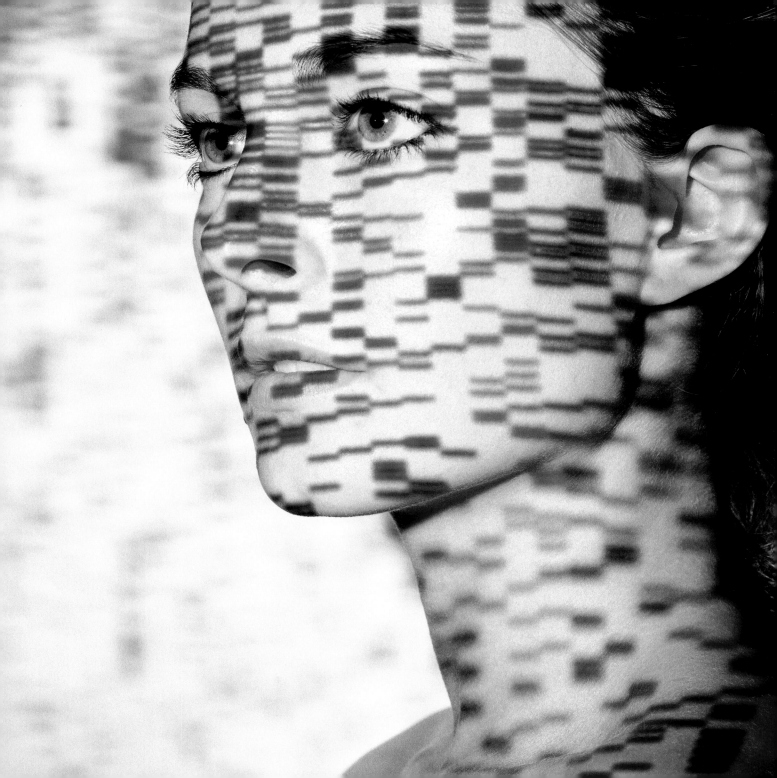

of women. This innate predisposition to cancer can be explained in part by the dizzying number of cell divisions required to form a human body consisting of 100,000 billion (10^{14}) cells originating from a single fertilized egg. With each of these divisions, cells have to copy all three billion letters in their DNA, a Herculean task that inevitably results in errors, or mutations, which occur spontaneously in certain genes essential for the overall equilibrium of these cells. The human body produces a million mutated cells every day, all with the potential to become cancerous. As a

result, even though cancer usually appears in adulthood, a great many of these mutations occur in the early years of our lives, between embryonic development and physical maturity (Figure 3). Even so-called identical twins, with exactly the same genes, accumulate mutations beginning in the embryonic growth phase and are therefore in many ways genetically distinct in adulthood.

These mutations mean that everyone — even people who are healthy — possesses a large number of abnormal cells that have, in some cases, evolved into microscopic tumors (Figure 4). For example, 50% of women in their forties have precancerous lesions in their breasts, and in 39% of women of this age, these lesions will already have reached the carcinoma stage, a proportion much higher than the incidence of this cancer in the population (15%). It is the same for pancreatic cancer: 74% of people have precancerous abnormalities in this organ, whereas this devastating cancer occurs in just 1.4% of the population. The remarkably high frequency of undetectable microscopic lesions, several times higher than the incidence of cancer in the population, thus indicates that we all have tumors inside us, but that in the majority of cases they remain hidden, invisible, like stowaways that can accompany us throughout our entire life without revealing themselves. In other words, we are biologically predisposed to cancer, but even more important, we are also predisposed to prevent full-blown cancer from occurring.

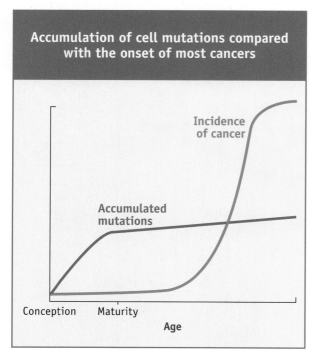

Accumulation of cell mutations compared with the onset of most cancers

Incidence of cancer

Accumulated mutations

Conception   Maturity

Age

Figure 3

Adapted from DeGregori, 2013.

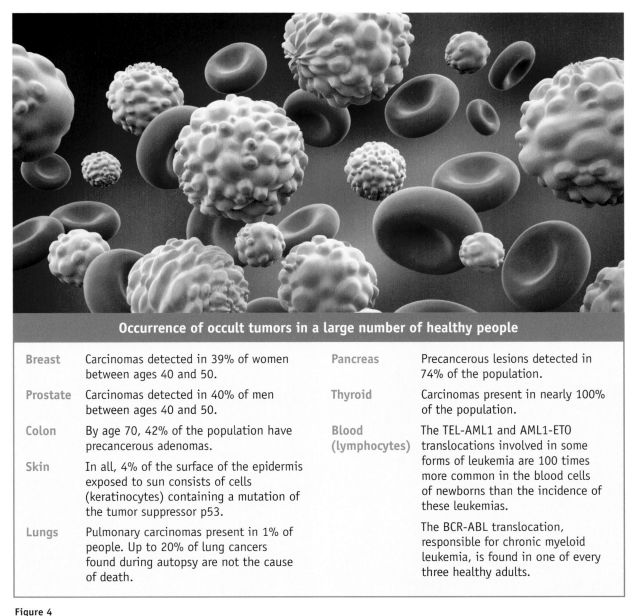

Occurrence of occult tumors in a large number of healthy people

Breast	Carcinomas detected in 39% of women between ages 40 and 50.	**Pancreas**	Precancerous lesions detected in 74% of the population.
Prostate	Carcinomas detected in 40% of men between ages 40 and 50.	**Thyroid**	Carcinomas present in nearly 100% of the population.
Colon	By age 70, 42% of the population have precancerous adenomas.	**Blood (lymphocytes)**	The TEL-AML1 and AML1-ETO translocations involved in some forms of leukemia are 100 times more common in the blood cells of newborns than the incidence of these leukemias.
Skin	In all, 4% of the surface of the epidermis exposed to sun consists of cells (keratinocytes) containing a mutation of the tumor suppressor p53.		
Lungs	Pulmonary carcinomas present in 1% of people. Up to 20% of lung cancers found during autopsy are not the cause of death.		The BCR-ABL translocation, responsible for chronic myeloid leukemia, is found in one of every three healthy adults.

Figure 4

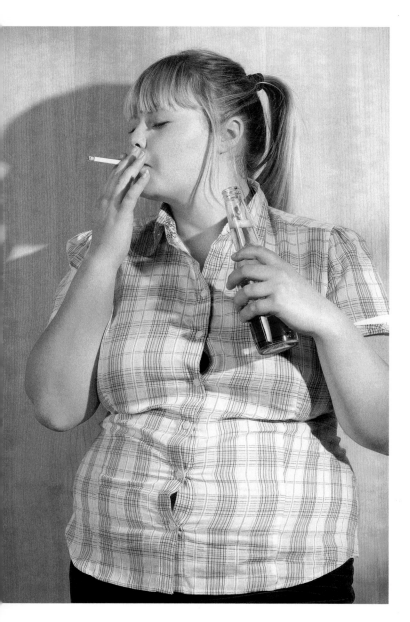

Bad Seed, Fertile Ground

Why do many spontaneously formed precancerous lesions remain latent in one person, and yet develop into cancer in another? Factors beyond our control, like aging and heredity, are often cited as the main agents determining cancer risk, but their influence is in fact much weaker than might be thought (see box).

Several studies indicate that it's really the major upheavals in lifestyle accompanying industrialization that have played a key role in providing precancerous lesions with optimal conditions for developing into cancer. For example, although our metabolism is adapted to a diet consisting mainly of plants, low in calories but high in fiber and antioxidant and anti-inflammatory compounds, current dietary habits are the exact opposite, based instead on the consumption of foods overloaded with sugar and fat, and therefore calories, while lacking plant- based protective molecules. As a result, two-thirds of the inhabitants of industrialized countries are currently overweight, with this accumulation of fat made worse by an unprecedented sedentary lifestyle, the result of technological progress that has radically decreased most people's energy expenditure. This way of life is conducive to the development of cancer: a bad diet, excess body weight and an overly sedentary lifestyle are all factors that can give an unexpected "boost" to precancerous cells

Not Just a Matter of Bad Luck

The high incidence of cancer is often viewed as a kind of "price to pay" for the increase in life expectancy that occurred in the last century. Yet age is clearly not the only factor in the equation, since the incidence of some cancers has risen in all age groups. Cancer of the esophagus has increased more than sixfold in the last 40 years, for all ages, and has now become one of the most rapidly increasing cancers (Figure 5).

Heredity plays a much less significant role than we might think, as attested to by the cancer risk in children adopted very early in their lives, one of whose biological or adoptive parents dies before age 50 of cancer. The death of an adoptive parent is associated with a very large increase in cancer risk in these children (500%), a proportion much higher than if a biological parent gets the disease (20%) (Figure 6). These children inherited their genes from their biological parents but got their lifestyle habits from their adoptive parents, suggesting that lifestyle factors are mainly responsible for cancer progression.

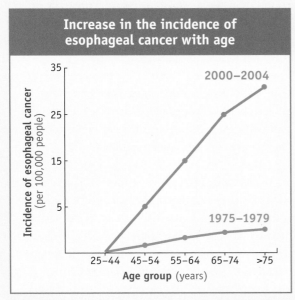

Increase in the incidence of esophageal cancer with age

2000–2004

1975–1979

Incidence of esophageal cancer (per 100,000 people)

Age group (years): 25–44, 45–54, 55–64, 65–74, >75

Figure 5 — Adapted from Brown et al., 2008.

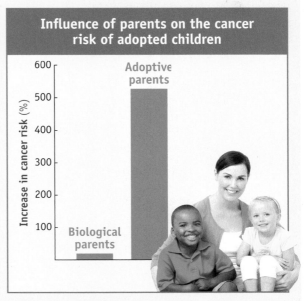

Influence of parents on the cancer risk of adopted children

Increase in cancer risk (%)

Adoptive parents

Biological parents

Figure 6 — Adapted from Sørensen et al., 1988.

by creating chronic inflammatory conditions that destabilize the body's normal equilibrium and promote cancer cell development.

Historically, inflammation has been associated with visible phenomena such as the sensation of heat, pain, redness, or swelling caused by a wound (the famous *calor*, *dolor*, *rubor* and *tumor* of Roman doctors). But chronic

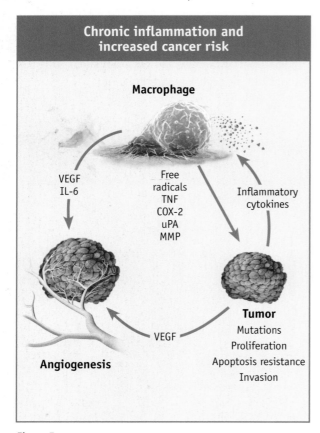

Chronic inflammation and increased cancer risk

Macrophage

VEGF
IL-6

Free
radicals
TNF
COX-2
uPA
MMP

Inflammatory
cytokines

VEGF

Angiogenesis

Tumor
Mutations
Proliferation
Apoptosis resistance
Invasion

Figure 7

inflammation is more insidious, since it develops without external signs and manages to severely disrupt the body's equilibrium. For example, chronic inflammation caused by obesity and a sedentary lifestyle is associated with increased production of oxygen and nitrogen free radicals that damage DNA and destabilize its structure. These radicals, as well as the messengers secreted by inflammatory cells located in the vicinity of tumor cells, can also compromise the functioning of some tumor suppressors (e.g., p. 53) and disrupt the delicate machinery whose job it is to repair DNA during cell division. At the same time, inflammatory cells secrete signals to recruit new blood vessels around the tumors so they can obtain the oxygen and nutrients they need for growth (Figure 7). In other words, chronic inflammation, whether it stems from a bad diet, too much fatty tissue, or physical inactivity, fundamentally changes the environment where precancerous cells are found, thus providing favorable surroundings for cells that have undergone mutations, or those containing epigenetic modifications essential for the progression of cancer, to emerge.

Cancer can thus be compared to a harmful seed that lies dormant inside each of us, but is only able to reach its full potential if it finds fertile ground to provide it with all the elements it needs to grow. And that's where the greatest paradox in our current approach to cancer lies: although we fear this disease and should do

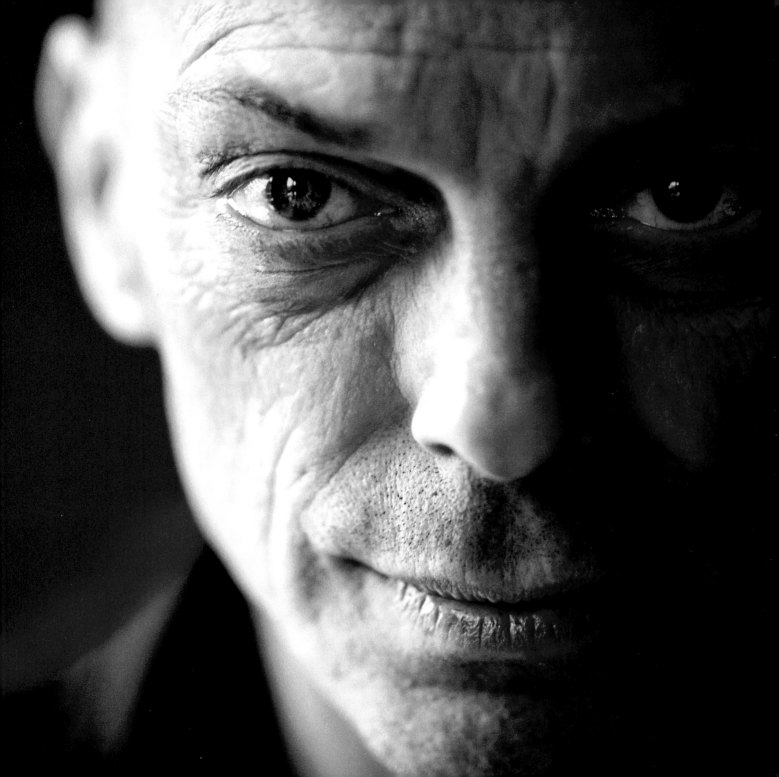

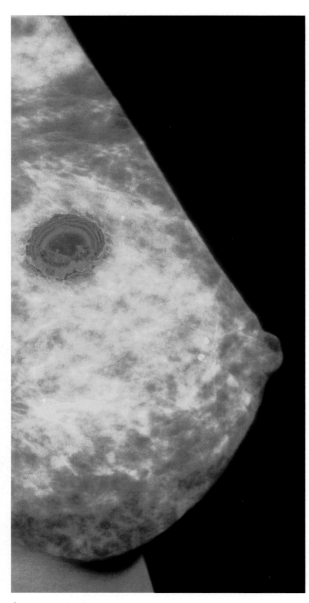

^ A tumor in the breast

everything we can to stop precancerous lesions before they become an uncontrollable force, our way of life makes their job easier by providing the favorable environment they need to reach their full destructive potential.

Cancers à la carte

Nothing better illustrates the harmful influence of the western way of life than the dramatic rise in the incidence of certain types of cancer among people who immigrate to the West. Women in China, Japan, Korea and the Philippines, for example, have among the lowest rates of breast cancer in the world, but this cancer can become up to four times more common among them after they immigrate to North America (Figure 8). This increase is a direct consequence of adopting a North-American lifestyle, with its high-calorie, low-plant diet, extremely sedentary habits and a marked increase in body weight. The impact of this way of life is such that the incidence of breast cancer among these immigrant women becomes similar to the incidence among American-born women by the third generation.

Even without emigrating, Asian women have seen their risk of breast cancer increase significantly in recent years, a consequence of the growing influence of the North-American lifestyle on all populations worldwide. In South Korea, for example, the incidence of invasive breast cancer has more than doubled in just 10 years, whereas mammary carcinomas in situ, an early form of cancer that appears in the walls of the milk ducts, through which milk flows to the nipple, have increased sixfold during this same period (Figure 9). The startling speed with which simple changes in lifestyle choices can increase the incidence of cancer indicates therefore that our daily habits — whether they be exposure to carcinogenic substances (tobacco, alcohol, ultraviolet rays), body weight, physical activity or diet — influence the functioning of the abnormal genes found in

microscopic tumors and can "wake up" these latent tumors, speeding up their progression to advanced stage cancer.

This interaction between genes and lifestyle habits is also observed in people with defective genes that predispose them to cancer. Women born with the BRCA1 gene mutation, for example, are at high risk of breast cancer, but the risk is now three times higher than at the beginning of the century. This appears to be a consequence of the excess calories in the modern diet and the marked increase in body weight seen in a growing number of people. Since the same phenomenon has been

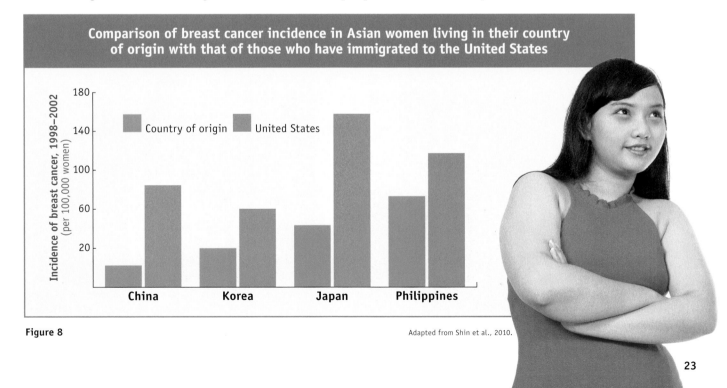

Comparison of breast cancer incidence in Asian women living in their country of origin with that of those who have immigrated to the United States

Incidence of breast cancer, 1998–2002 (per 100,000 women)

Country of origin ■ United States

China — Korea — Japan — Philippines

Figure 8

Adapted from Shin et al., 2010.

observed in carriers of another mutation that increases the risk of breast cancer (BRCA2), we can conclude that even when there is a serious genetic predisposition known to encourage the development of cancer, our modern-day lifestyle remains the most influential risk factor for getting the disease.

Taming Cancer

Our current approach to cancer must therefore be completely rethought: cancer that has reached an advanced stage and can be clinically detected is actually an anomaly, a form that has very little in common with what a cancer really is for most of its "lifetime" inside the body. In the span of a human life, it's very unlikely that a cancer cell can simply acquire by chance all of the mutated genes it needs to develop into cancer. To reach a mature stage, a cancer has to be able to count on the collaboration of its surroundings, on changes in the prevailing anti-cancer environment that normally prevents it from acquiring the properties it needs to develop further. In some animals, this anticancer environment is so restrictive that it succeeds in completely preventing the development of any kind of cancer (see box)! Obviously, this is not

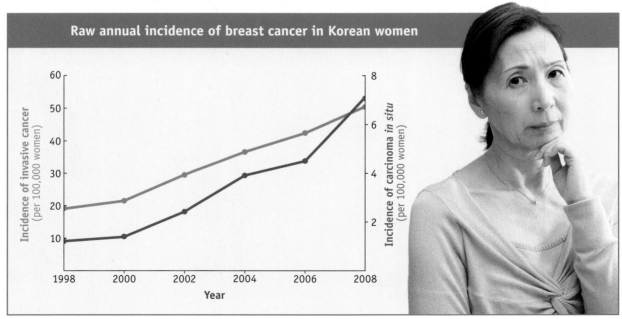

Figure 9

Adapted from Jung et al., 2011.

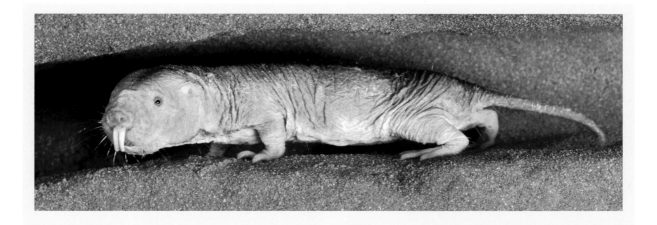

Why Does the Mole Rat Never Get Cancer?

The naked mole rat (*Heterocephalus glaber*) is a very unusual African rodent, both because of its disconcerting appearance and its way of life, similar to that of social insects like ants or bees (eusociality). The most fascinating aspect of this animal is its ability to live for a very long time and in excellent health: whereas rodents of its size usually live for 4 or 5 years, the mole rat can live for nearly 30, which corresponds to nearly 600 years for a human being! This exceptional longevity is due to the animal's innate resistance to the main illnesses that normally accompany aging, including cancer.

The mole rat seems to owe this total absence of cancer to the extreme elasticity of its skin, a physiological adaptation that allows it to move quickly through the underground tunnels it digs to reach the roots and tubers it feeds on. Fibroblasts, the cells of the connective tissue surrounding cells, secrete a special form of hyaluronic acid, a viscous substance that welds the cells together, creating a kind of jelly that makes the skin very flexible. Since the connective tissue coating the cells is the first barrier that cancer cells have to break through to implant themselves in a particular tissue, the hyaluronic acid creates an environment resistant to tumor growth. Even when very aggressive cancer cells are injected into the animal, they are unable to implant themselves and are quickly eliminated. The mole rat thus shows the degree to which an organism's natural defenses can influence the risk of getting cancer.

the case for human beings, but our defenses are nonetheless effective enough to slow down the progression of precancerous cells and make cancer an extremely drawn-out process, during which an abnormal cell has to overcome a great many obstacles to reach a stage where it is advanced enough to invade the organ that has sheltered it for several years (Figure 10).

In terms of prevention, therefore, making the most of this very long latency period is essential in order to tame the disease, live with it and ensure that the microscopic precancerous lesions, made up of several thousand cells, never undergo the many mutations needed to become a mature cancer: nine mutations for breast cancer, 11 for colon cancer and 12 for prostate cancer. People who adopt healthy lifestyle habits deprive these microscopic tumors of several elements indispensable to their growth, thus encouraging these immature cancers to remain in a latent state. On the other hand, repeated exposure to carcinogenic substances (tobacco, alcohol, ultraviolet rays) and the creation of a chronic inflammatory environment through poor lifestyle choices creates conditions that

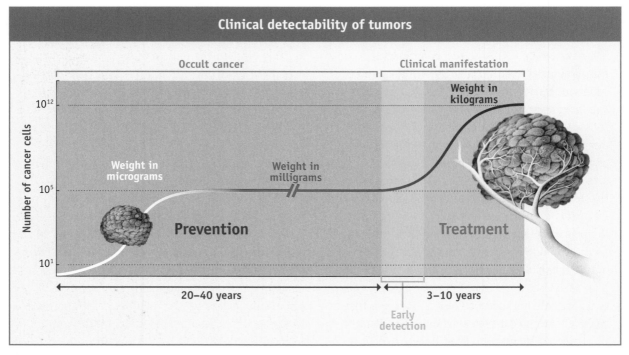

Figure 10

Adapted from Almog, 2013.

Tracking Down Fugutives

One of the most encouraging advances in cancer research in recent years is the advent of increasingly reliable methods of detecting, at an early stage, tumors that have managed to avoid the body's natural defense systems. Current anticancer treatments are much more effective when used against small tumors. Early detection of these tumors has therefore considerably improved the prognosis for some cancers, as shown in the significant decrease in mortality from colorectal cancer in several western countries, a success attributable to colonoscopy programs. For breast and prostate cancers, the benefits of screening are less certain, as many tumors that are detected early are in fact benign cancers that would not have progressed during the patient's lifetime. The considerable decline in patients' quality of life associated with the treatment of these tumors then becomes a problem, since they would not have been life-threatening even if they had remained undetected. That said, despite the risks of overdiagnosis and overtreatment inherent in all forms of large-scale screening, the possibility of detecting a tumor as early as possible is considered the best option currently available for treating cancer. And it's important for people at risk to participate in existing screening protocols. It must be understood, however, that early detection of a tumor is only a complement to cancer prevention. A detectable tumor already

has several million very unstable cells with a large number of mutations that can cause them to develop into a mature cancer or resist chemotherapy. Aggressive treatment may make it possible to eliminate these tumors, but the intervention will not automatically be successful. It's still much better to prevent cancer by halting its evolution at the source, before it reaches the size where it can be detected by current technology.

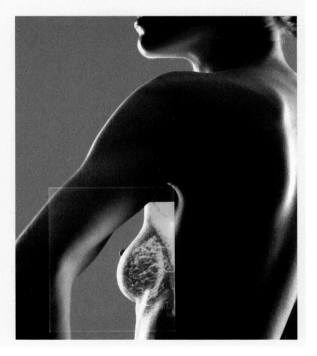

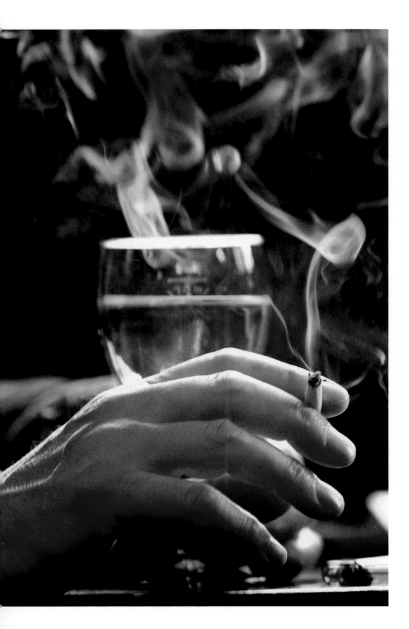

aid the development of these microtumors and the growth of a cancerous mass made up of several million cells. There is nothing abstract or theoretical about this concept. For example, although the Japanese have an incidence of prostatic microtumors similar to that among western men, these precancerous lesions develop more slowly in Japan than in the West, meaning that the clinical symptoms and mortality linked to prostate cancer are 10 times lower in Japan than in North America. On the other hand, these differences have diminished considerably in recent years, owing to the adoption of a western lifestyle by the Japanese. Cancer prevention therefore does not so much mean preventing cancer cells from appearing inside the body, but rather delaying their progression long enough to keep them from reaching a mature cancer stage during the eight or nine decades of a human lifespan. Although these precancerous lesions are benign, their development can quickly take a tragic turn: a cancerous lesion that has managed to conquer these natural defense systems contains several thousand mutated cells whose highly unpredictable behavior poses a serious threat to the body. The fastest possible detection of these tumors using screening techniques then becomes essential to increase the likelihood that the therapeutic arsenal will be able to eradicate them (see box p. 27).

Preventing Cancer

There is therefore no reason to be defeatist with respect to cancer. On the contrary, the potential for preventing this disease is quite remarkable: it's estimated that only about 25% of all cancers are the result of random mutations alone (Figure 11), and that mortality related to cancer could be significantly reduced in the coming decades, if we choose to devote the major part of our efforts to the prevention and early detection of the disease.

This preventive approach is even more realistic given that research in recent years has made it possible to identify the broad outlines of what must be done to significantly reduce the risk of developing several kinds of cancer, particularly those that hit the populations of industrialized countries especially hard (lung, breast, colon and prostate). The first step is to reduce exposure to toxic agents like cigarette smoke, alcohol and ultraviolet rays. These agents all have the ability to attack DNA directly and to introduce excess errors that increase the likelihood of mutations occurring in several genes essential for controlling cell growth. Repeated exposure of organs in close contact with these carcinogens (the lungs to tobacco, the oral cavity to alcohol and skin to ultraviolet rays) thus facilitates the malignant progression of cells, as attested to by the increase in cancer risk in these organs (from 10 to 40 times) in people with these lifestyle habits.

That said, most people do not smoke, they drink alcohol in moderation, and they do not expose themselves needlessly to

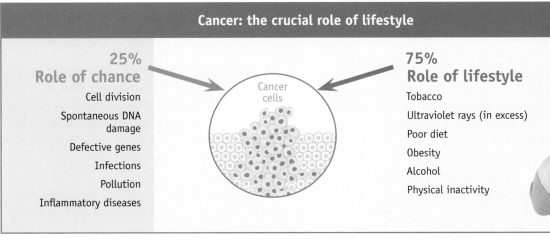

Cancer: the crucial role of lifestyle

25%
Role of chance

Cell division

Spontaneous DNA damage

Defective genes

Infections

Pollution

Inflammatory diseases

Cancer cells

75%
Role of lifestyle

Tobacco

Ultraviolet rays (in excess)

Poor diet

Obesity

Alcohol

Physical inactivity

Figure 11

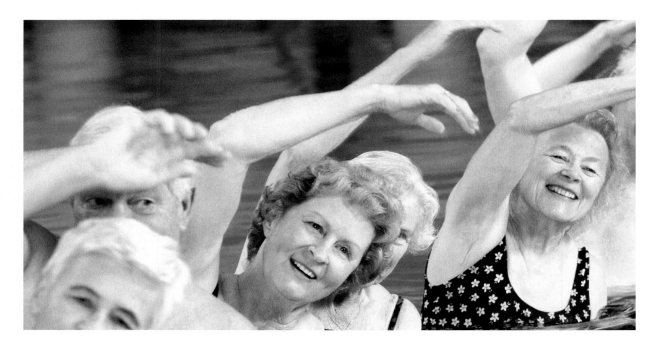

the sun; yet many of these people will still get cancer as a result of the effect of other lifestyle habits on the environment where cancer cells are found. In this vein, a host of studies have shown beyond any doubt that three of the main lifestyle aspects currently widely observed in industrialized countries contribute to the high incidence of cancers in these populations: (1) the accumulation of too much fat, especially when it goes above a certain threshold and leads to obesity; (2) a poor-quality diet consisting mainly of products with too many calories and not enough fiber, minerals and plant-based phytochemical compounds; and (3)

our extremely sedentary modern societies, the collateral damage of automation and technological progress in general.

Thanks to the outstanding work of a number of public health agencies, notably the World Cancer Research Fund and the American Cancer Society, current knowledge about cancer prevention can be summarized in the form of 10 major recommendations (Figure 12).

These recommendations are the result of a rigorous evaluation of several hundred thousand studies by the greatest experts in cancer research, and as such represent one of the most important achievements in cancer research in recent decades. The main goal of this book is to explain in simple terms the scientific discoveries that have led to these recommendations, to enable readers to better understand, on the one hand, the degree to which each of these habits can influence cancer risk and, on the other, the need to change some aspects of their lifestyle to reduce this risk. This approach is all the more important since prevention is not part of western culture, which is focused on short-term rather than long-term benefits; in addition, prevention usually runs counter to the financial interests of multinational corporations, which are trying to promote the consumption of their products — be these tobacco, carbonated beverages or over-processed foods stripped of essential nutrients — with no concern for their negative impact on the health of the population (Figure 13).

The positive impact of following these recommendations has been studied in recent years, and the results are remarkable. For example, a recent study involving menopausal women indicates that following at least five of these recommendations is related to a 60% reduction in the risk of invasive breast cancer (Figure 14). Similar results have

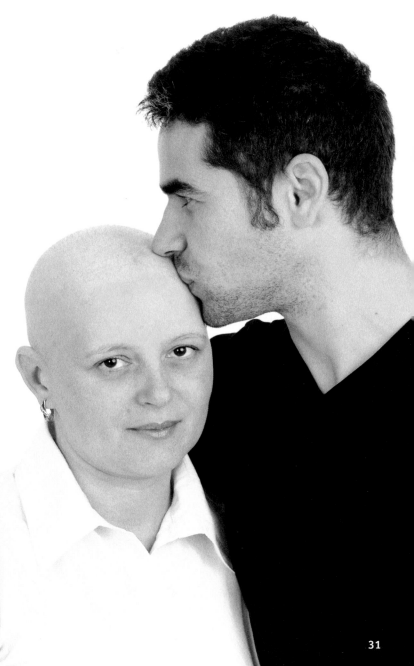

The 10 main recommendations for preventing cancer

		Main cancers involved
	1. Stop smoking. All tobacco products are harmful to health.	Lung Bladder Pancreas
	2. Stay as lean as possible, with a body mass index of between 21 and 23. Avoid carbonated beverages and limit as much as possible the consumption of energy-dense foods containing large quantities of sugar and fat.	Colon Breast Endometrium
	3. Limit the consumption of red meat (beef, lamb, pork) to approximately 1 lb (500 g) per week, replacing it with meals based on fish, eggs or vegetable proteins.	Colon Breast Pancreas
	4. Eat more of a variety of fruits, vegetables and legumes, as well as foods based on whole grains. These foods should make up two-thirds of a meal.	All
	5. Be physically active at least 30 minutes every day.	Colon Breast

Figure 12

Main cancers involved

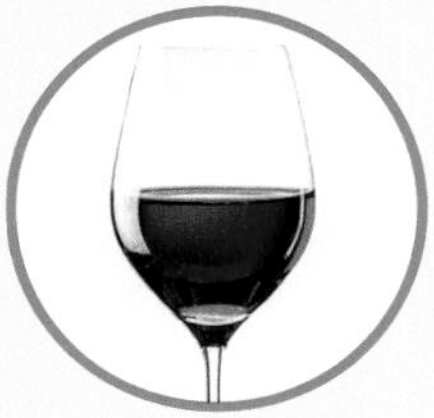

6. Limit daily alcohol consumption to two glasses for men and one for women.

Oral cavity
Breast

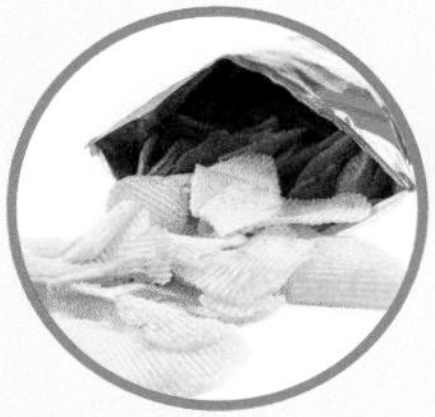

7. Limit consumption of products preserved with salt, as well as products containing large amounts of salt.

Stomach

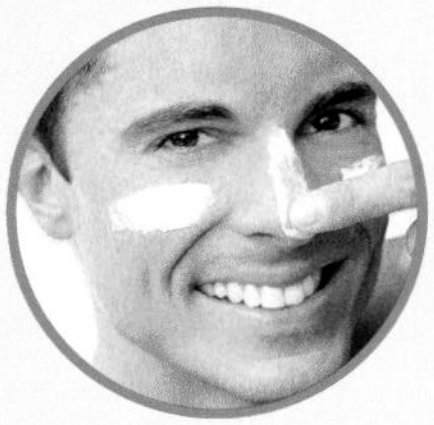

8. Protect the skin by avoiding unnecessary sun exposure. When it's impossible to remain in the shade, wear protective clothing or apply sunscreen.

Skin

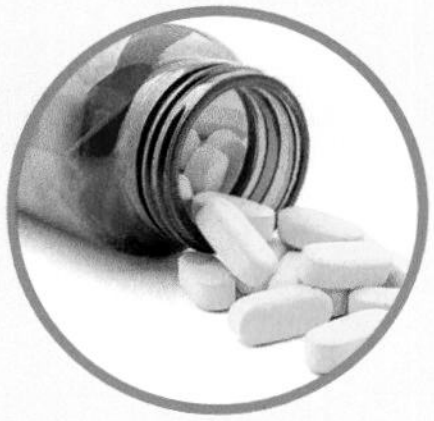

9. Don't use supplements to protect against cancer: studies clearly show that the synergy of a combination of foods is by far superior to supplements for decreasing the risk of cancer.

All

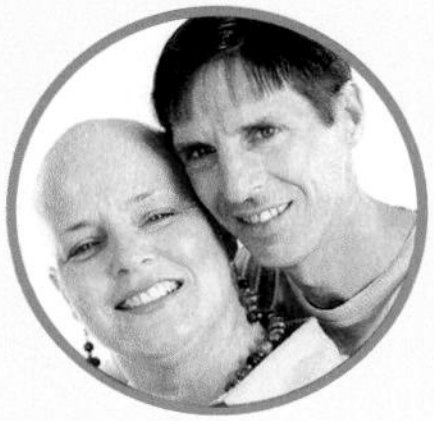

10. Cancer survivors should follow the above recommendations, to the letter.

All

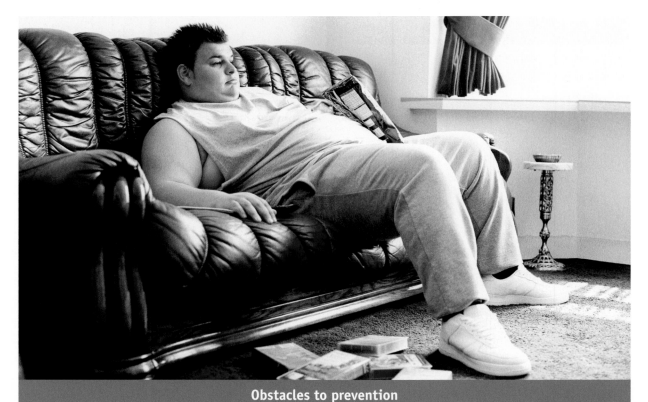

Obstacles to prevention

- Success is not visible.
- These lifestyle changes are "boring" and difficult to maintain.
- The "average lives" documented by statistics are not very motivating to people.
- It usually takes a long time for benefits to become apparent, whereas people expect benefits in the short term.
- Behavior change must be long-term — in other words, permanent.
- People take risks even when these could be avoided.
- Commercial interests run counter to prevention of the disease.
- Some advice may be in conflict with personal, religious or cultural beliefs or values.

Figure 13

Adapted from Fineberg, 2013.

been reported for breast cancer survivors and for men with prostate cancer, illustrating how much these recommendations can influence the mortality caused by cancer.

It is absolutely imperative that we make the most of these discoveries, in order to reverse the current trend and finally progress in our fight against cancer. And, as we will see in the following chapters, this preventive approach is much less complicated than we might think.

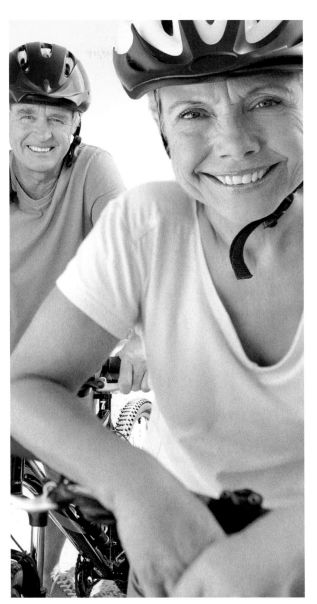

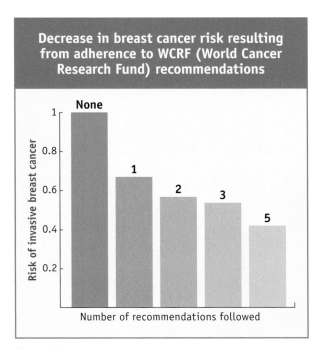

Decrease in breast cancer risk resulting from adherence to WCRF (World Cancer Research Fund) recommendations

Figure 14   Adapted from Hastert et al, 2013.

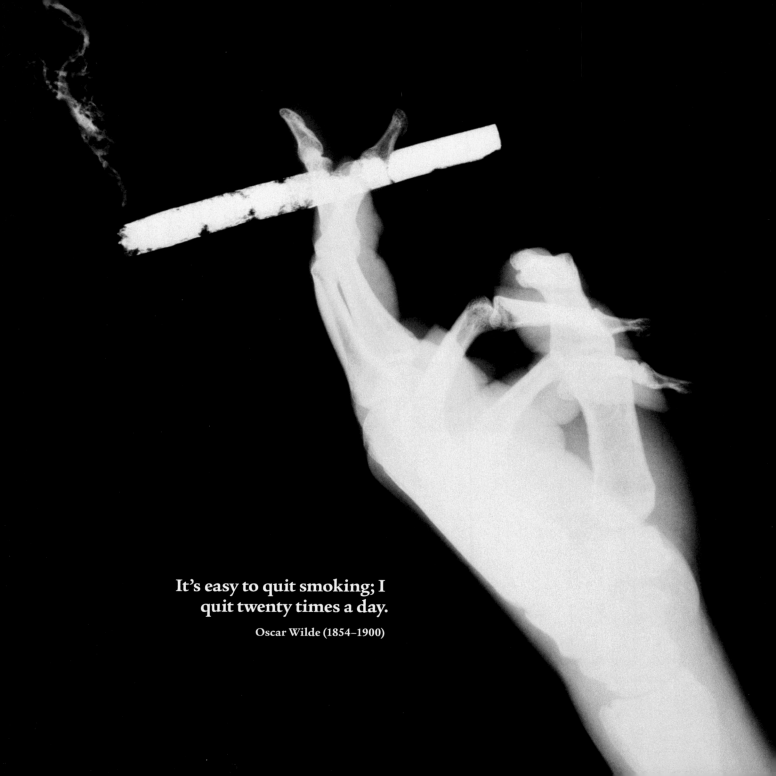

It's easy to quit smoking; I
quit twenty times a day.

Oscar Wilde (1854–1900)

Chapter 2

Tobacco: A Smoke Screen for Cancer

Recommendation
Quit smoking.

Source: American Cancer Society

In the majority of cultures, smoke has always been considered sacred, the symbol of the spirit rising to the heavens to communicate with the gods, enabling us to honor the dead and purify or protect the living. These smudging ceremonies were very important in the Native American tradition, especially those that involved burning tobacco, a sacred plant believed to have been at the origin of the creation of the universe. Native to the American continents, where about 60 wild species still grow, tobacco has been used for millennia by many Native American tribes as a fundamental element in a large number of religious and social — even shamanic — rituals, to communicate with spirits. Tobacco held such an important place in Native American life that when Christopher Columbus landed in the Bahamas and Cuba in 1492, one of the Taïnos' first acts was to offer him dried tobacco leaves as a gift and to invite him to smoke *tobagos* with them, a kind of tobacco leaf tube through which they inhaled smoke into their mouths or noses. This first contact was to have incalculable consequences later on, as many of Columbus's companions adopted these customs enthusiastically and, on their return home, introduced smoking to the European continent.

Although smoke rituals held religious and symbolic meaning for Native Americans, Europeans quickly discarded these spiritual meanings for more "down to earth" considerations. Some, like French diplomat Jean Nicot, believed tobacco possessed curative qualities; he even succeeded in persuading Catherine de' Médici to use it to soothe the migraines of her son, Francis II. Tobacco use spread rapidly among the aristocracy, mainly in the form of a powder to be inhaled; its popularity earned Nicot the privilege of seeing the *Nicotiana tabacum* plant named in his honor. But it was really the "recreational" side of sniffing or smoking that remained the main motivation for tobacco users; many people agreed that "There is nothing to be compared with tobacco; it is the passion of all people of quality; and he that lives without tobacco is not fit to live." (Molière, *Don Juan*, 1665; translation Curtis H. Page, 1908). As a result, despite energetic efforts by some to contain the spread of tobacco (see box), the sacred herb of the Americas reserved for solemn occasions gradually became a commonly consumed substance, cultivated and exported all over the world.

Yet it was not until the end of the 20th century, with the invention of automated machines able to make large quantities of cigarettes, that tobacco use really took off and spread throughout the entire population. For example, whereas Americans in 1870 smoked on average less than one cigarette (0.36) per person per year, this number had risen to 1,485 by 1930, and eventually reached a peak of 4,259 cigarettes in 1965. A resounding commercial success, no doubt, but also one that triggered an unprecedented health crisis, with more than 100 million people in the 20th century dying from cancer, cardiovascular disease and lung disease caused by smoking. And this crisis is far from over, as tobacco consumption continues to rise, with approximately 6,000 billion cigarettes now smoked worldwide every year, the equivalent of roughly 1,000 cigarettes for every man, woman and child on the planet (Figure 15). At this rate, it is predicted that smoking will be directly responsible for a billion deaths in the 21st century.

Tobacco dependency is not usually the result of a conscious and informed choice by smokers, but is actually the outcome of large-scale manipulation cleverly orchestrated by the tobacco industry to make, promote and

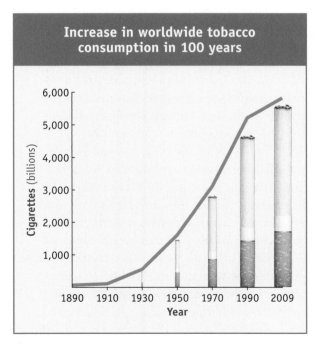

Increase in worldwide tobacco consumption in 100 years

Figure 15   Adapted from www.tobaccoatlas.org, 2010.

Where There's Smoke ...

Although tobacco spread like wildfire all over the world, its use did not gain anything like unanimous support. Rodrigo de Jerez, Christopher Columbus's companion, who took the first "cigars" to Spain, was denounced by his neighbors, who were frightened to see him exhaling smoke through his nose and mouth, and thrown in prison by the Inquisition for demonic practices. For James I of England, tobacco use was a habit "loathsome to the eye, hateful to the Nose, harmefull to the braine, dangerous to the lungs." He even went so far as to decapitate Sir Walter Raleigh, whom he reproached (among other things) for having brought the plant from Virginia to Great Britain. A number of rulers in the Middle East, Europe and Asia were not exactly thrilled about this new habit either: the Chinese emperor Ming Chongzhen, the last of his dynasty, declared war on tobacco by threatening to decapitate anyone who imported or used it. As for Persia's Shah Abbas I the Great, he had the nose cut off of anyone who took snuff and mutilated the lips of smokers, whereas his close neighbor, the Ottoman sultan Murad IV, had them burned alive on a pyre of tobacco leaves. Even the Russian czar Alexis I, despite being called the "very peaceful czar" because of his open mind and clemency, ordered that a smoker caught in the act be condemned to death or have his nose cut off.

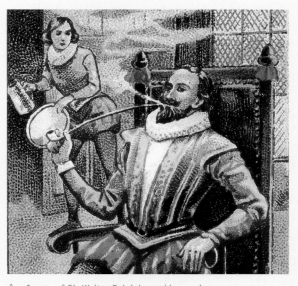

^ Image of Sir Walter Raleigh smoking a pipe

As awful as they were, these punishments were nonetheless powerless to eradicate the spread of tobacco, and tobacco users continued to risk their lives to obtain the precious herb. Governments had the last word, however, and in the end most countries established monopolies for the sale of tobacco that would allow them to make considerable profits from their citizens' addiction. These governments would in turn become dependent on the income from tobacco, which explains in large part why tobacco is still sold over the counter, despite the 100 million or so deaths directly linked to its use during the 20th century.

legitimize products that it well knows to be very harmful. For the cigarette as we know it today is not just a paper tube full of tobacco — it is a very sophisticated industrial product carefully developed to maximize the potential for dependence on one of the plant world's most addictive substances: nicotine.

A Devastating Insecticide

Nicotine is in fact an alkaloid with a powerful insecticide action used by a number of plants in the Solanaceae family as a defense mechanism against insects. Mainly found in tobacco, nicotine is also present in other species within this family — tomatoes, peppers, eggplant, potatoes — but in much smaller amounts. For example, you would have to eat 22 pounds (10 kg) of eggplant or 375 pounds (170 kg) of peppers to get the dose of nicotine in one cigarette (Figure 16)! It's also interesting to note that these low doses of nicotine in foods could have positive effects on health, notably by decreasing the risk of getting Parkinson's disease.

Nicotine is found in very large amounts in the leaves of the tobacco plant, from which it can even evaporate and spread to neighboring plants, thus eliminating nearby insects. There is so much nicotine in tobacco that when the leaves are wet, people harvesting them can be exposed in a few hours to massive doses of

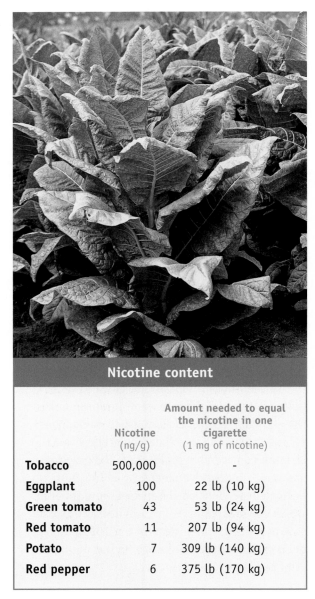

Nicotine content

	Nicotine (ng/g)	Amount needed to equal the nicotine in one cigarette (1 mg of nicotine)
Tobacco	500,000	-
Eggplant	100	22 lb (10 kg)
Green tomato	43	53 lb (24 kg)
Red tomato	11	207 lb (94 kg)
Potato	7	309 lb (140 kg)
Red pepper	6	375 lb (170 kg)

Figure 16   Adapted from Henningfield, 1993.

nicotine equivalent to smoking roughly 50 cigarettes, which can cause dizziness, vomiting, headaches and muscle weakness. This "green tobacco sickness" is especially dangerous for children employed in some countries as a workforce to harvest tobacco for American multinationals, with disastrous consequences for their physical and mental development.

Nicotine's molecular structure resembles that of acetylcholine, a neurotransmitter used by nerve cells to transmit nerve impulses, and can activate this transmitter's so-called nicotinic receptors. Large doses of nicotine thus cause excessive stimulation of the neural circuits, just like other toxic agents that increase acetylcholine levels, such as organophosphorus insecticides or poison gases like sarin. There is nothing pleasant about nicotine poisoning, with its combination of nausea, vomiting, excessive salivation, difficulty in breathing, irregular pulse and convulsions that quickly cause death.

Nicotine Dependence

How can a molecule as toxic as nicotine create dependence, the irrepressible need smokers experience to keep smoking despite all of its known negative consequences? One of the basic principles of pharmacology is that the dose makes the poison, and nicotine is a good

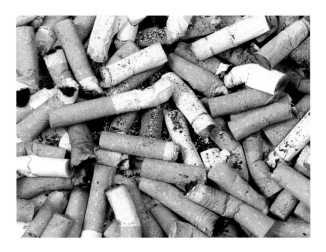

example of this. Although high amounts of this drug overstimulate the neural circuits and can cause death, nicotine that is inhaled, and is therefore present in lower doses, specifically activates certain neurons in the nucleus accumbens, a tiny region in the brain that plays a major role in what is called the "reward circuit" (Figure 17). When nicotine activates these neurons, dopamine, a neurotransmitter that signals a pleasant experience — a source of pleasure — is released, immediately giving the act of smoking a "positive" connotation. Inhaled nicotine is also found in all parts of the body, but it has only a weak interaction with the nerve cells governing muscle movement. In a way, this is too bad, for if tobacco caused intolerable and possibly fatal muscle contractions, smoking could never have seen the light of day.

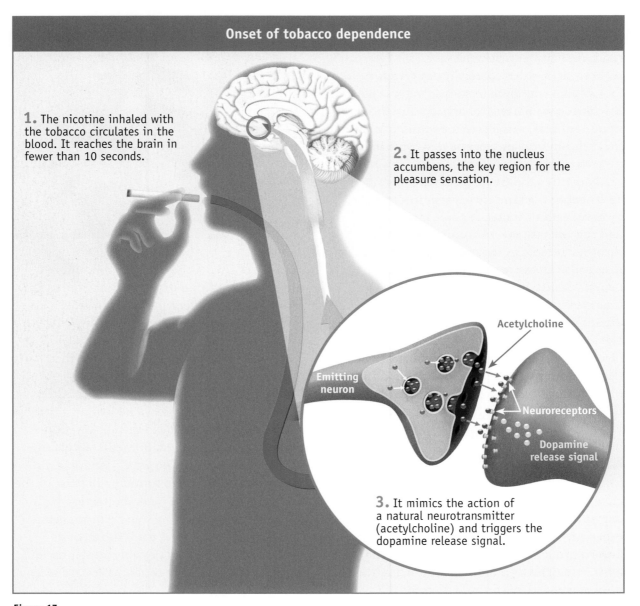

Onset of tobacco dependence

1. The nicotine inhaled with the tobacco circulates in the blood. It reaches the brain in fewer than 10 seconds.

2. It passes into the nucleus accumbens, the key region for the pleasure sensation.

Acetylcholine

Emitting neuron

Neuroreceptors

Dopamine release signal

3. It mimics the action of a natural neurotransmitter (acetylcholine) and triggers the dopamine release signal.

Figure 17

The creation of this reward circuit is obviously not instantaneous; for most people, the first cigarette just causes a cough or nausea, effects that are far from pleasant! However, in people who repeat the experience and begin to smoke regularly, brain function is gradually changed, "reprogrammed" little by little, so that the reward circuit activated by nicotine is slowly reinforced and becomes increasingly important for the person's feeling of well-being. At the same time, certain molecules in cigarette smoke increase dopamine levels by blocking the enzymes (monoamine oxidases) that control its degradation, creating a synergy with nicotine that heightens the reward effect associated with smoking. This circuit thus causes very powerful dependence — more than a third of people who have smoked at least one cigarette become tobacco dependent — which makes nicotine the most addictive substance on the market (Figure 18).

Yet there is nothing "recreational" about being dependent on tobacco, when compared to the use of other drugs; smoking a cigarette induces neither euphoria, hilarity nor a feeling of ecstasy. The pleasure or anti-stress effect that smokers associate with the act of smoking is actually just relief from the cravings experienced by people used to tobacco. This dependence imposes a number of constraints on smokers, for although nicotine acts almost instantaneously, reaching the brain less than

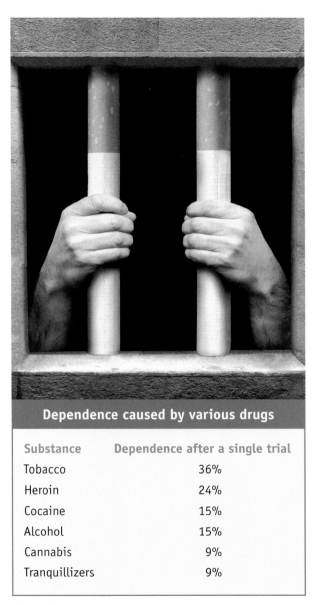

Dependence caused by various drugs

Substance	Dependence after a single trial
Tobacco	36%
Heroin	24%
Cocaine	15%
Alcohol	15%
Cannabis	9%
Tranquillizers	9%

Figure 18

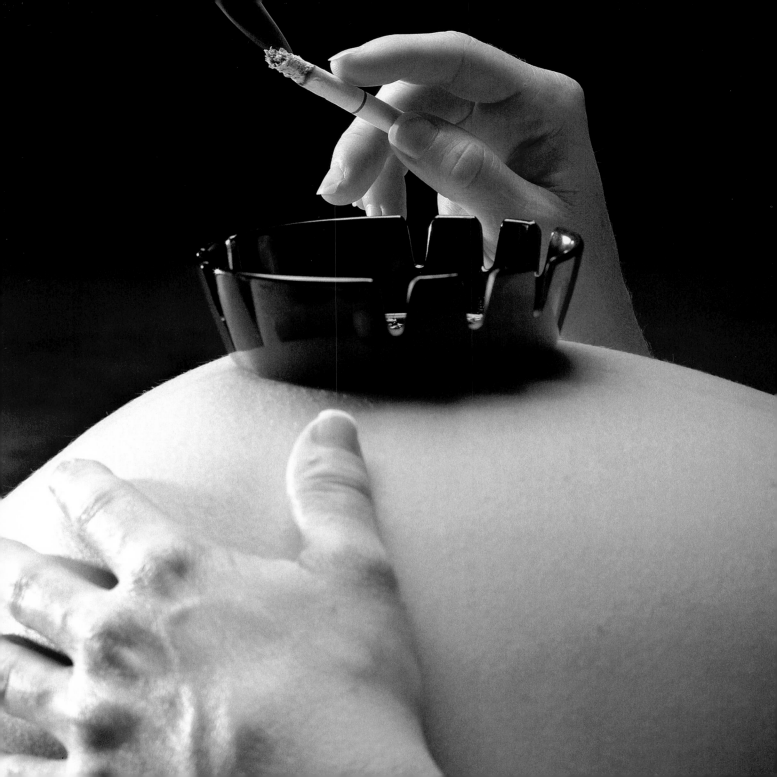

10 seconds after cigarette smoke is inhaled, its effect dissipates quickly. People who are dependent must therefore smoke frequently to maintain enough nicotine in their blood and avoid cravings. Generally speaking, at least 10 to 20 cigarettes are needed to reach this goal, and barely 8% of smokers manage to smoke fewer than five cigarettes a day, without ever smoking more. Smokers also have a remarkable ability to regulate on their own the amount of nicotine they take in to maintain their "nicotinemia" at a high enough level by inhaling more deeply the smoke from the first cigarettes of the day, or from those smoked before entering the office or during a break, for example. Studies also indicate that smokers of cigarettes that used to be called "light," containing less nicotine, inhale more frequently and more deeply to make up for the decrease, which at the same time increases the absorption of the harmful substances in cigarette smoke.

The main motivation for a tobacco-dependent person is not therefore to experience an altered or ecstatic state, but really to avoid the feelings of discomfort caused by a lack of nicotine. Smoking is not like drinking alcohol; it's more like being alcoholic, a kind of slavery that literally poisons one's existence. Furthermore, many surveys show that most people who are dependent on tobacco would like to quit smoking or have even tried to do so several times without success, because of their inability to deal with the cravings that go along with nicotine withdrawal.

Creating Dependence

Today's cigarettes have very little in common with the tobacco smoked by Native Americans or by the first European colonists who settled in the Americas. Traditionally, tobacco leaves were dried in the open air, producing a bitterly pungent brown tobacco (like the tobacco in cigars, for example) that

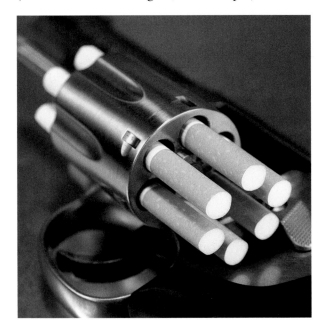

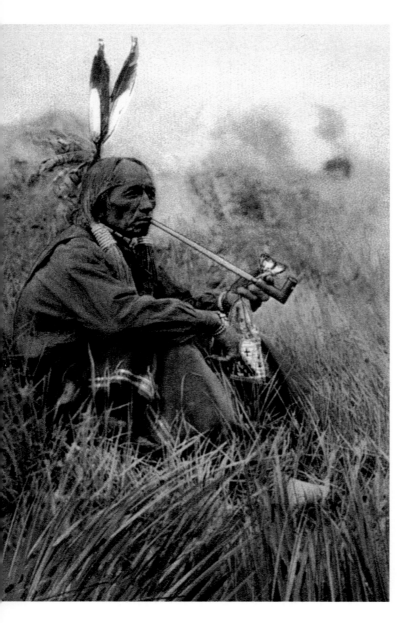

was almost impossible to inhale deeply because of the irritation of the respiratory tract caused by its smoke. These smokers thus absorbed limited amounts of nicotine, mainly in the oral cavity, and physical dependence on tobacco was, as a result, less pronounced than it is today. With the invention of a new method of drying tobacco leaves using heat (flue-curing) toward the end of the 19th century, cigarettes really became addictive. This technique caused major biochemical changes in the plant's leaves that yielded a milder and sweeter yellow tobacco whose smoke could be deeply inhaled, causing the absorption of larger amounts of nicotine through blood circulation in the lungs. Armed with this "new generation" tobacco, American cigarette companies would succeed in conquering the world, finding a way to use every occasion, even tragic ones, to portray cigarettes as a "modern" and attractive product (see box).

The most appalling aspect of the history of cigarettes, however, remains the tobacco industry's relentless efforts to make smokers as dependent as possible. This conspiracy, brought to light by the documents in the *Master Settlement Agreement* (see box p. 48), clearly shows that this industry spared no effort to increase the amount of nicotine inhaled by smokers, with the admitted objective of increasing their dependence on cigarettes. For example, American cigarette manufacturers

Tobacco Wars

The two world wars played a determining role in the staggering increase in cigarette consumption in the 20th century. Whereas at the beginning of the century cigarette smoking was considered to be a habit of effeminate men — "real" men chewed tobacco or smoked cigars — manufacturers capitalized on the Americans' entry into the war in 1917 to provide cigarettes at low cost to "support the troops' morale." A gesture appreciated by an American general of the day, John Pershing, according to whom, "to win this war [soldiers needed] tobacco as much as bullets," but the result of which was nonetheless that millions of men who had never smoked came back from the front inveterate smokers. Cigarettes had gained a new respectability and barely 20 years later, in 1939, 66% of American men aged 40 or under smoked regularly.

The end of the World War II would give tobacco manufacturers another opportunity to sell their products more widely, this time to the European population as a whole. Because of the insistence of a senator from Virginia, influenced by the local tobacco industry, roughly one billion dollars' worth of cigarettes was sent to Europe under the Marshall Plan, representing nearly 10% of the total amount destined for the reconstruction of Europe. This American tobacco was much milder than the brown and very bitter tobacco in fashion in Europe at the time, which meant that smokers could inhale more deeply, absorb larger amounts of nicotine and, in turn, quickly become dependent on cigarettes. The tobacco industry had thus managed to benefit from the two biggest crises to have shaken humanity in the 20th century to dramatically increase sales of its products, a feat that turned these companies into financial giants, but at the cost of catastrophic repercussions for people's health.

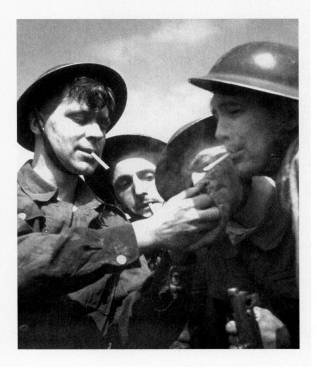

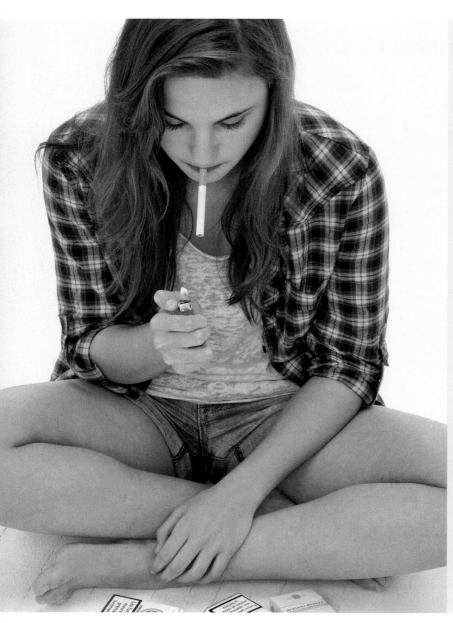

Smoking Documents

The *Master Settlement Agreement* is a 1998 agreement entered into by the four main American tobacco companies (Philip Morris Inc., R.J. Reynolds, Brown & Williamson, and Lorillard) and the attorneys general of 46 American states, who sued these tobacco companies for reimbursement of healthcare expenses related to smoking. The result was not a conviction, but just a friendly agreement establishing that these businesses had to pay the states $206 billion over 25 years. But in addition to the financial issues, the judges ruled that internal memos, confidential reports and research results accumulated over the preceding 50 years by the industry had to be released. The publication of these tobacco documents, totaling more than 85 million pages, made it possible to penetrate the industry's secrets and divulge its efforts to make cigarettes more addictive, its activities to fight back against anti-tobacco activists, its plans for marketing to teenagers and its diversionary tactics for fooling the public by instilling doubt as to the results of studies on the harmful effects of cigarettes.

add 616 chemical products to tobacco, some of which aim to make the smoke easier to tolerate, whereas others are expressly designed to increase the availability of nicotine and make it easier to absorb. Adding ammonia, for example, makes smoke more alkaline and allows nicotine to be converted into a more easily assimilated chemical substance, a process similar to that used to change cocaine into crack, an alkaline form of the drug, which is absorbed more quickly and creates greater dependence. Adding sugars sweetens the taste of tobacco and generates, as it burns, acetaldehyde; this leads to the formation of monoamine oxidase inhibitors that increase the levels of dopamine and dependence on tobacco. Even substances like menthol, added to reduce irritation caused by smoke, encourage dependence by increasing the number of acetylcholine receptors in the brain, which causes a smoker to consume more cigarettes. These chemical manipulations have definitely had an impact on the toxicity of cigarette smoke, for between 1968 and 1985, the concentrations of carcinogenic agents like 2-naphthylamine and 4- (methylnitrosamino)-1-(3-pyridyl)-1-butanone (NNK) increased by 59% and 44%, respectively. Cigarette companies thus continued to make and promote products that aimed to keep smokers dependent, with no regard for the impact on their health, even though they were perfectly aware of the dangers of smoking. This capitalism without scruples is not just accidental, for

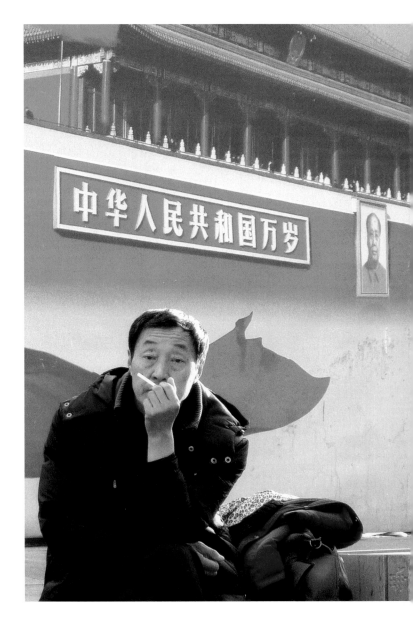

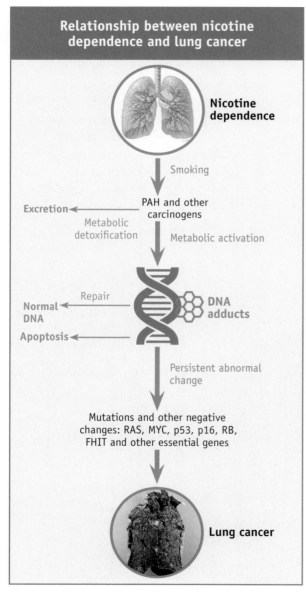

Relationship between nicotine dependence and lung cancer

Nicotine dependence

↓ Smoking

PAH and other carcinogens

Excretion ← Metabolic detoxification

Metabolic activation ↓

Repair
Normal DNA ←
Apoptosis ←

DNA adducts

↓ Persistent abnormal change

Mutations and other negative changes: RAS, MYC, p53, p16, RB, FHIT and other essential genes

↓

Lung cancer

Figure 19   Adapted from Hecht, 1999.

even though the dangers of tobacco have been scientifically proven beyond a doubt, the tobacco industry has persisted in its practices and profited from opening up new markets like China, India, Russia, Indonesia and Africa to sustain its growth and reap staggering profits. Furthermore, these are now the regions with the highest proportion of smokers; for example, 60% of men in East Timor and Indonesia and 50% of Russians are dependent on cigarettes. The tobacco industry's expansionist aims, along with a growing world population, have resulted in a significant increase in the number of smokers worldwide in the last 25 years.

A Weapon of Mass Destruction

By manipulating tobacco to increase its addictive properties, the tobacco industry has created what may be the most devastating weapon in the history of humanity. Not because of nicotine absorption, since nicotine has no major impact on health in small doses, but rather because dependence on tobacco means that smokers are repeatedly exposed to several carcinogenic molecules in cigarette smoke. Polycyclic aromatic hydrocarbons (PAHs) and some nitrosamines, for example, are especially dangerous, as these molecules are metabolized into highly reactive compounds that attach themselves directly to cell DNA and can cause mutations. Every pack of cigarettes is thought to contain enough carcinogenic compounds to cause two DNA mutations in lung cells, which means that decades of smoking result in the accumulation of several thousand of these mutations, increasing the risk of cancer when they occur in genes that are key to controlling cell growth (Figure 19). The link between smoking and lung cancer is clearly shown by the marked rise in the incidence of this cancer following increased consumption of cigarettes in the first half of the 20th century. Once an extremely rare disease, this cancer started to become more and more common 20 years or so after the introduction of cigarettes and has

not stopped increasing since (Figure 20). The long latency period between starting to smoke and getting lung cancer is a good illustration of how slowly cells become cancerous, even in the presence of a substance as carcinogenic as tobacco. The absence of harmful effects in the short term also explains in part why smoking was able to become so widespread in large segments of the population, including among health professionals, as smokers simply could not have suspected that continuous exposure to tobacco contributed to the inexorable development of cancer.

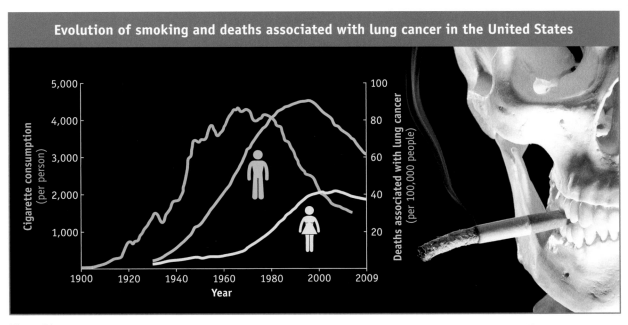

Figure 20

Adapted from www.cancer.org, 2013.

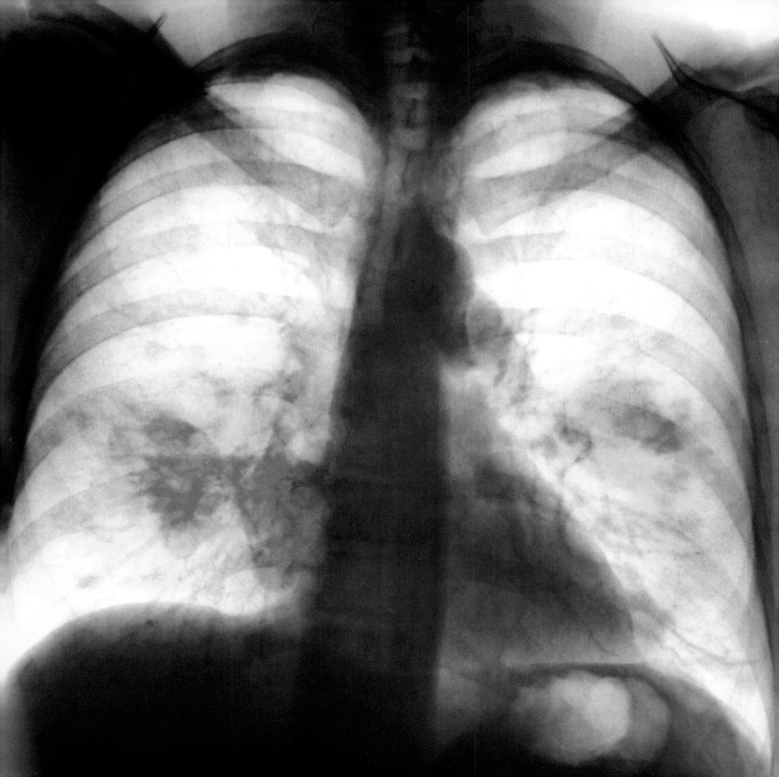

Cigarette smoke contains at least 3,500 different compounds, several of which contribute to smoking-related lung cancer. For example, a tobacco plant has the strange property of incorporating polonium 210, a radioactive isotope formed from the decomposition of the uranium in the earth's crust, into its leaves. Although present in tiny amounts, the polonium 210 is absorbed with each puff of a cigarette and gradually accumulates in the respiratory tract, so that someone who smokes a pack of cigarettes a day is exposed in just 1 year to radiation equivalent to 300 x-rays of the thorax. Polonium, 250 million times more toxic than cyanide, was actually used to murder ex-KGB agent Alexander Litvinenko, then in exile in London.

In addition to the lungs, several other organs are exposed to the carcinogens in tobacco, and at least 10 different types of cancer are associated with smoking (Figure 21).

The upper digestive system (mouth, larynx, pharynx and esophagus), which is directly in contact with cigarette smoke, is an obvious target for carcinogens, but other internal organs are also at high risk. For example, smokers are two or three times more likely to develop bladder cancer, since their urine contains elevated amounts of carcinogenic aromatic amines like

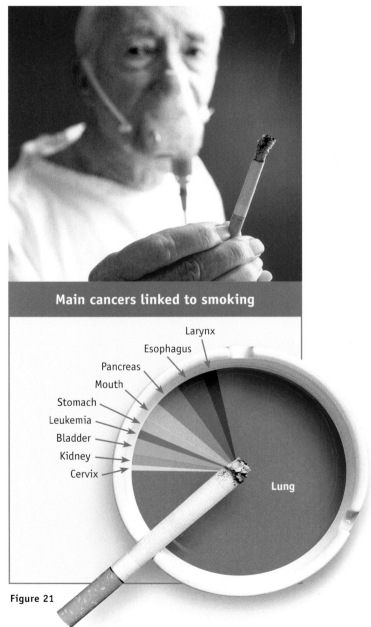

Main cancers linked to smoking

Larynx
Esophagus
Pancreas
Mouth
Stomach
Leukemia
Bladder
Kidney
Cervix
Lung

Figure 21

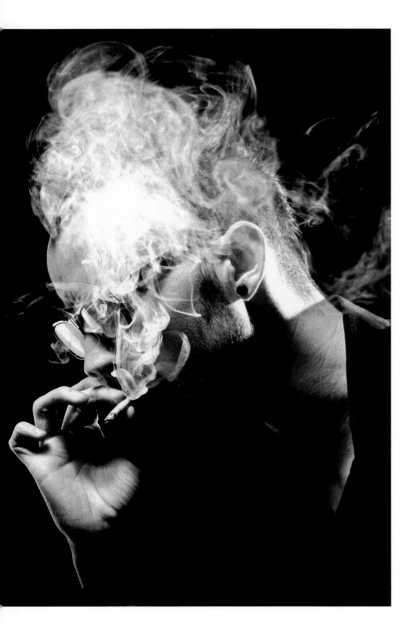

2- naphthylamine and amino-4-diphenyl, which cause significant DNA damage in the cells of the bladder lining. Bladder cancers related to smoking have increased dramatically in recent years, another likely consequence of the greater absorption of carcinogens caused by deeper inhalation of cigarette smoke.

Because of all of these factors, combined with the negative impact of tobacco on the functioning of several organs, especially the respiratory and cardiovascular systems, smoking is associated with a dramatic decrease in life expectancy, with people who smoke throughout their adult lives dying 10 years earlier than nonsmokers, on average.

Breaking the Chains

The well-documented effects of tobacco on health have aroused vigorous reactions from public health agencies in almost every country. Large-scale information campaigns, a sizable increase in tobacco taxes, banning publicity and prohibiting smoking in public spaces have all contributed to a significant decrease in the percentage of smokers worldwide, which has gone from 41% in 1980 to 31% in 2012 for men, and from 11% to 6% for women. In countries like Canada, Norway and Iceland, this decrease is even more dramatic, although roughly 20% of the population still smokes.

Quitting smoking is hard, but these considerable decreases in tobacco use show that millions of people have done it, most without assistance. Even nowadays, when many anti-smoking aids are available, the vast majority of people who stop smoking do so by themselves, without pharmacological or psychological assistance. Nicotine substitutes or drugs like bupropion (Zyban) or varenicline (Champix) can be helpful and increase the cessation success rate by about 50%, but there is nothing miraculous about them: the motivation to quit is still the main factor in successfully abstaining from tobacco use.

Given this, is it possible to further reduce the number of die-hard smokers or those who can't seem to stop? This is a delicate question, for if such a large number of people continue to smoke despite the exorbitant cost of cigarettes and the regulations against smoking in all public spaces and in many homes (one-quarter of smokers do not smoke in their own homes), current coercive approaches will likely soon reach their limits. Some aspects of laws can be improved by banishing tobacco from public outdoor spaces, for example, but if we exclude prohibition (because of the risk of the boomerang effect observed during alcohol prohibition), it's difficult to imagine how society could impose an even more restrictive environment on smokers. Given the highly addictive nature of nicotine, the only way to really reduce smoking in the longer term is to prevent a new clientele from experiencing the taste of tobacco.

To make this happen, we first have to remember that the tobacco companies have absolutely no scruples about the catastrophic effects of their products on health and are determined to sell them no matter what the cost.

In this kind of environment, young people are a prime target for cigarette companies, and recent years have witnessed the very aggressive

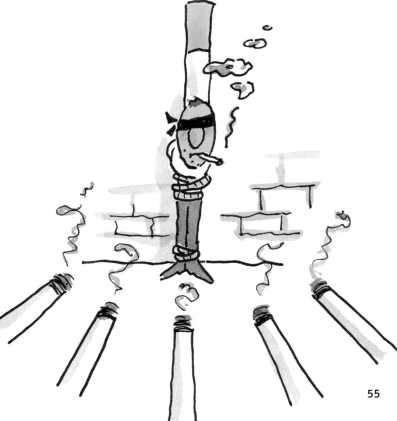

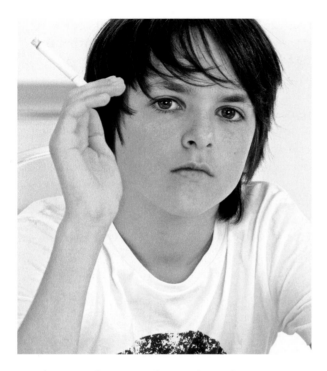

dimension to the fight against tobacco (Figure 22). The principle at the root of these products is relatively simple: a solution of nicotine in glycerin or propylene glycol is heated with an atomizer, which creates a white vapor that looks like cigarette smoke. The "e-smoker" thus inhales a small amount of nicotine, like a smoker, but the vapor does not contain the many carcinogenic molecules and fine particles formed by burning tobacco. These products are essentially vehicles for administering a drug, nicotine, but are far less dangerous than traditional cigarettes, both in terms of cancer and heart and lung disease.

The use of e-cigarettes has been greeted with enthusiasm by many health professionals who deal daily with the ravages of tobacco. According to them, this is a valid strategy for reducing the damage caused by cigarettes, an approach that targets consequences rather than behaviors, somewhat in the way syringe exchange programs for drug addicts are used to reduce the risk of AIDS or hepatitis.

Recent studies indicate that e-cigarettes increase the likelihood of successful smoking cessation by 60%, suggesting that these products are not only alternatives to tobacco, but could also prove to be useful tools for quitting smoking. For opponents of any form of smoking, on the other hand, e-cigarettes are a kind of Trojan horse, a springboard to

marketing of new products whose flavors (chocolate, mint, cherry, candy) are clearly designed to attract young adults. Because this industry is incapable of regulating itself and continues to promote products with disregard for the consequences for the health of the population, the only way to put an end to this influence is to change current laws so as to ban all flavored tobacco products, including those with menthol.

The arrival on the market of the electronic cigarette, or "e-cigarette," could also add a new

bringing tobacco back into the mainstream that could reverse the gains made in recent years. It is obviously essential to strictly regulate the marketing and sales of these products, especially among young people, so as to reduce as much as possible their exposure to this toxic substance; recent studies also indicate that e-cigarette vapor contains high levels of nanoparticles that stimulate inflammation and increase the risk of asthma, heart disease and diabetes. Nonetheless, the decreased

damage associated with replacing current cigarettes with their electronic version cannot be rejected out of hand, especially for people who are dependent on nicotine and unable to quit. Every year, six million people die from diseases caused by cigarettes, and the gradual elimination of traditional tobacco products could mark a major turning point by preventing millions of premature deaths in the 21st century.

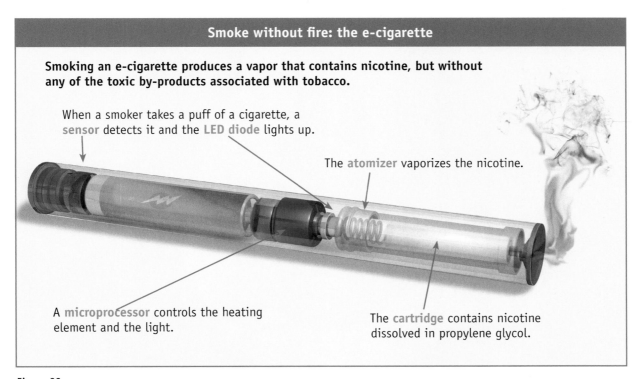

Smoke without fire: the e-cigarette

Smoking an e-cigarette produces a vapor that contains nicotine, but without any of the toxic by-products associated with tobacco.

When a smoker takes a puff of a cigarette, a **sensor** detects it and the **LED diode** lights up.

The **atomizer** vaporizes the nicotine.

A **microprocessor** controls the heating element and the light.

The **cartridge** contains nicotine dissolved in propylene glycol.

Figure 22

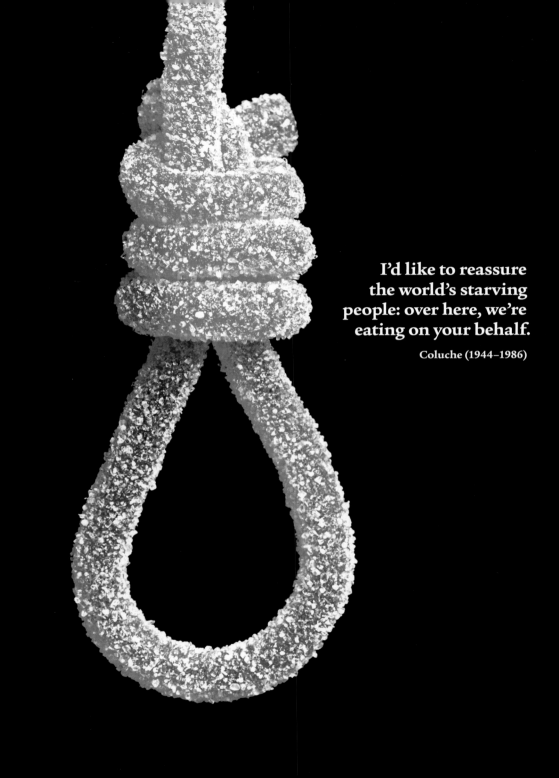

I'd like to reassure
the world's starving
people: over here, we're
eating on your behalf.

Coluche (1944–1986)

Chapter 3

An Expanding Universe

Recommendation
Stay as lean as possible, with a body mass index (BMI) of between 21 and 23. Avoid carbonated beverages and limit as much as possible the consumption of energy-dense foods containing large quantities of sugar and fat.

Source: World Cancer Research Fund International

In recent decades, a multitude of products overloaded with fat, sugar, salt and refined flours, but lacking in many essential nutrients, have literally invaded public space and resulted in an unprecedented change in people's dietary habits. These foods, whether they are carbonated beverages, snacks and candy, frozen meals or other "modern" products made by food multinationals, are very often strictly industrial creations, a mixture of purified ingredients (fat, sugar, salt, various additives) that have been cleverly assembled to create attractive products, easy to use and able to be preserved for long periods. The biggest revolution brought about by these processed industrial products, however, has been to concentrate the energy in food at levels never before seen, several times higher than in naturally sourced foods. A plain candy, swallowed in barely a few seconds, is a veritable energy bomb containing more calories than a complete meal, whereas a simple fast-food meal eaten on the go, sometimes even in the car, can meet an entire day's caloric needs on its own. The impact of this industrialization of food has been remarkable: whereas barely a century ago these products did not exist, they now make up more than 75% of food sales worldwide.

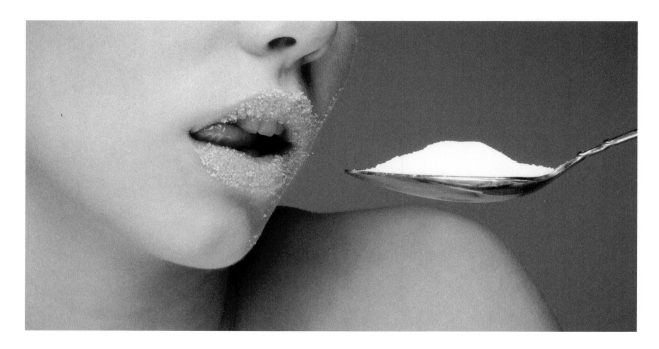

An Optimal Sensory Experience

The high calorie content of industrial food products is not the only thing that makes these foods popular. Sugar and fat are energy sources essential for survival, and we are biologically attracted to these substances, but it would not cross anybody's mind to eat the roughly 10 spoonfuls of sugar in a can of pop straight from the sugar bowl, nor to drink the four spoonfuls of cooking oil in a small bag of chips. The reason many of these industrial products are so appealing is because they have actually been carefully designed to create

an "optimal sensory experience," the most favorable brain reaction possible in response to the taste, look and texture of these foods. This has been a resounding success, with several studies clearly showing that just looking at high- sugar, high-fat industrial foods is enough to activate the parts of the brain involved in the reward circuit and responsible for the pleasure sensation. A study done using magnetic resonance imaging, a technology that makes it possible to visualize brain activity in real time, has even shown that a single spoonful of ice cream is enough to stimulate these parts of the brain! The industrial foods that abound in our environment are thus anything but harmless; they are actually highly complex products whose nutritional inadequacy is masked by excess sugar and fat combined in such a way as to create a unique brain "experience" that encourages their consumption.

Artificial Paradises

Several rodent studies have clearly established that the activation of the brain's reward circuits by sugar and fat is very similar to that brought about by some drugs. For example, animals given the choice between a sugary drink and an intravenous dose of cocaine prefer the sugar. Similarly, animals that have free access to fatty foods like sausages, bacon or cheesecake quickly become dependent on these kinds of food; this addiction is characterized by their compulsive consumption, even when eating them is associated with electric shocks. This dependence on fat is also accompanied by a tolerance for these foods resulting in decreased production of dopamine, responsible for the pleasure sensation, which causes animals to eat even more to make up for this hedonic deficiency. A lower reward response has also been observed in humans who eat ice cream frequently, with this tolerance leading to subsequent overconsumption of the food to obtain the sought-after satisfaction. Since loss of control and substance tolerance are

well-known characteristics of drug dependence, several researchers have put forward the theory that the extra sugar and fat in modern industrial foods might be addictive and create a dependence in some people similar to that associated with drug use.

Calories for Sale

In contrast to drugs, food is essential for life, and it's difficult to establish precisely just how much dependence is caused by the repeated consumption of high-calorie foods. What we can safely affirm is that the food industry itself is completely dependent on these products, without which it cannot hope to maintain its grip on our dietary habits. Nor is it accidental that this industry devotes considerable efforts to targeting young people through publicity, toys and product placement; this

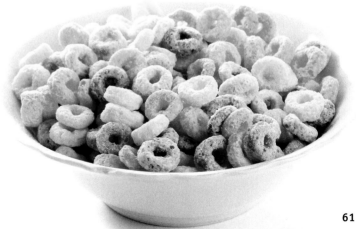

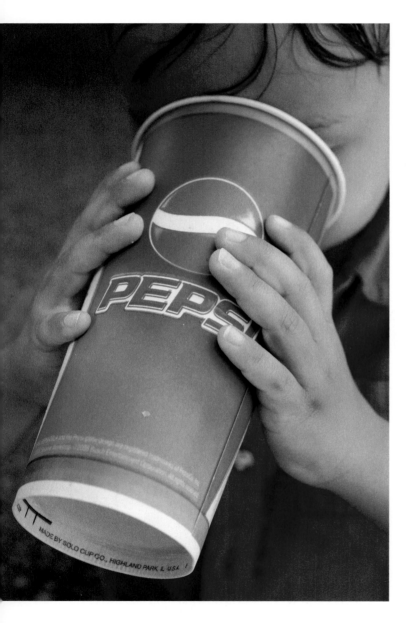

is a deliberate ploy to earn the loyalty of a whole new generation of consumers as early as possible, by influencing from childhood their taste for fatty and sugary foods. Highly processed industrial foods must therefore not be viewed as a perfectly normal food source, but as the merchandise they are — products for consumption made from low-quality, cheap ingredients, but which, because of their caloric attractiveness and very aggressive marketing, are successfully sold on a large scale and generate staggering profits. In North America, barely 10 or so food giants control over half of food sales, and it must never be forgotten that the main objective of these multinationals is to post profitable growth for their directors and shareholders, even if that means marketing products of mediocre nutritional quality. And whether we like it or not, just as with the cigarette industry, the corporate interests of these companies are incompatible with consumers' health.

Caloric Overload

The immediate impact of the proliferation of highly processed industrial foods has been to significantly increase the quantity of calories consumed by the population (Figure 23). In the United States, for example, the massive influx of these products, beginning in the 1980s, has been accompanied by a gradual rise in calorie intake, which reached a peak of 2,700 kcal per day per person by the year 2000, an increase of 25% compared with barely 20 years earlier.

Since the level of physical activity has remained unchanged during this period, the extra energy intake has obviously had major repercussions on the body weight of the population: 70% of people are currently overweight (BMI > 25) — compared with 50% of the population in 1980 — and 34% of these are actually obese (BMI > 30), almost three times more than 30 years ago (Figure 24).

Sugar's pervasiveness in the modern industrial diet is the main culprit in the consumption of excess calories. Whereas sugar used to be an ingredient used almost exclusively in desserts or other small occasional treats, it's now estimated that 80% of the 600,000 or so currently available food products contain added sugars. Sugar is found almost everywhere, in cereals, snacks, bread, salad dressings, sauces and yogurts, especially when these products are billed as low fat: a plain 0% fat vanilla-flavored yogurt can contain as many as 5 teaspoons of sugar, half of what is in a can of pop! We are therefore exposed daily to enormous amounts

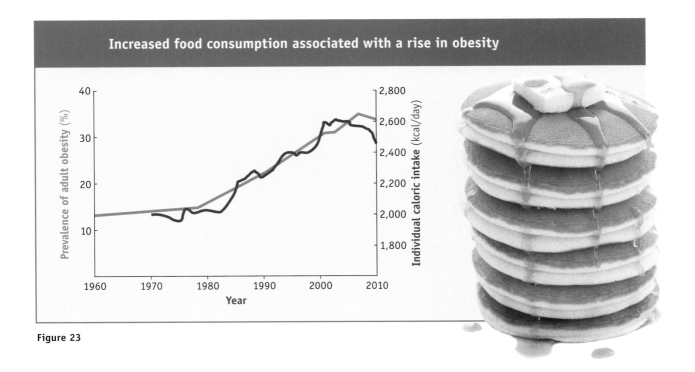

Increased food consumption associated with a rise in obesity

Figure 23

Too Much Sugar

The sugar added to industrial foods is mainly in the form of sucrose (table sugar) or corn syrup with added fructose (high fructose corn syrup, or HFCS). In both cases, these sugars are formed by combining a molecule of glucose and a molecule of fructose: what we call sucrose is a sugar composed of 50% glucose and 50% fructose, whereas HCFS contains 45% glucose and 55% fructose. Although HFCS is a purely industrial product and may seem to be more harmful than "natural" table sugar, these two sugars are biochemically similar and thus have identical effects on the body.

Consuming too much sugar is harmful to health, as it overloads the mechanisms that maintain glucose and fructose concentrations at levels compatible with the body's proper functioning. An amount of glucose that exceeds energy needs, for example, is converted to fat and then deposited in the fatty tissue, which over time leads to an increase in body mass. Managing excess fructose is even more difficult, since our system does not have what it needs to deal with this substance, which accumulates in the liver where it's changed into fat. (This is actually the process used to create foie gras, by force-feeding geese or ducks with corn as a source of fructose.) These physical responses to too much sugar can in the long run cause major metabolic disturbances, notably the onset of chronic hyperglycemia that can lead to type 2 diabetes.

Carbonated beverages offer perhaps the best illustration of the harmful effects associated with consuming too much sugar. These drinks, just like their modern cousins (energy or sports drinks, vitamin waters, various juice-based cocktails), are really caloric "bombs" that can contain almost 3½ tablespoons (40 g) of sugar in every can. They are very popular with young people and can make up as much as 15% of their daily calorie intake. Several studies have clearly shown that consuming these drinks is associated with weight gain, one reason being that calories absorbed in liquid form do not cause a feeling of fullness and are therefore consumed in addition to those in food. Similarly, the excess fructose that comes from the absorption of sugary foods, like carbonated drinks, seems to upset liver function and cause serious blood lipid disorders, a risk factor for heart disease, not to mention that recent studies suggest that some cancer cells might prefer fructose for growth.

The discovery of sweeteners (aspartame and sucralose [Splenda], for example) revolutionized the soft drink industry, since it allowed manufacturers to offer consumers products deemed "healthier," with no sugar and therefore no calories. This is, however, just an illusion, as several studies have shown that the impact of these drinks is similar to that of standard soft drinks — in other words, increased risk of obesity, type 2 diabetes, heart disease and metabolic syndrome. Currently available data suggest that the brain does not like us fooling it with "fake sugars" containing no calories: sugar is essential for the brain to function, and a lack of calories causes a state of "dissatisfaction" characterized by less activation of the brain's reward centers, which are usually stimulated by sugar. The brain then reacts by stimulating the appetite for other sweet foods to make up for the sweeteners' lack of calories, which can result in excess caloric intake. Soft drinks, whether they are diet or not, are actually bad foods that disrupt our metabolism and promote the development of serious chronic diseases that reduce life expectancy. There is therefore no reason to consume these drinks regularly, even to quench thirst.

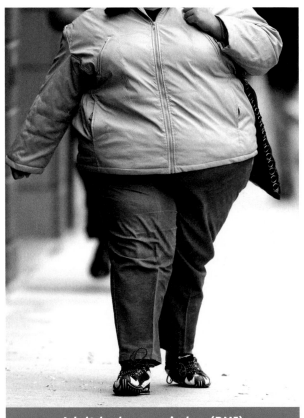

Adult body mass index (BMI)	
BMI	Category
18.5–24.9	Normal weight
25–29.9	Overweight
30–39.9	Obesity
40 +	Morbid obesity

BMI is calculated using the equation
$BMI = $ weight in kg/(height in m^2).

Figure 24

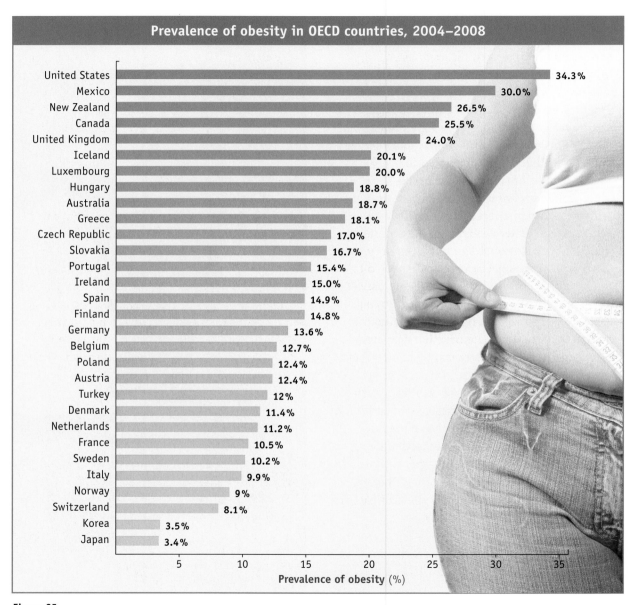

Prevalence of obesity in OECD countries, 2004–2008

Country	Prevalence of obesity (%)
United States	34.3%
Mexico	30.0%
New Zealand	26.5%
Canada	25.5%
United Kingdom	24.0%
Iceland	20.1%
Luxembourg	20.0%
Hungary	18.8%
Australia	18.7%
Greece	18.1%
Czech Republic	17.0%
Slovakia	16.7%
Portugal	15.4%
Ireland	15.0%
Spain	14.9%
Finland	14.8%
Germany	13.6%
Belgium	12.7%
Poland	12.4%
Austria	12.4%
Turkey	12%
Denmark	11.4%
Netherlands	11.2%
France	10.5%
Sweden	10.2%
Italy	9.9%
Norway	9%
Switzerland	8.1%
Korea	3.5%
Japan	3.4%

Prevalence of obesity (%)

Figure 25

of sugar, often in spite of ourselves, and some researchers maintain that this increased consumption could be at the root of the rapid increase in the proportion of the population that is overweight observed in recent years (see box p. 65).

Obesity without Borders

Although Americans are unquestionably the "heavyweight" champions of the world, inhabitants of other countries have also seen their size increase considerably in recent years (Figure 25). Trade globalization has led to the spread of a vast array of industrial processed foods all over the world, and every country, without exception, that has adopted these new food habits has to deal with a greater proportion of obese individuals. The rapid increase in consumption of high-calorie industrial products in countries in economic transition is especially disturbing in this respect, as the resulting increase in obesity coexists in many cases alongside food insecurity and malnutrition in these populations.

The ready availability and low cost of highly processed foods allow poor people to meet their energy needs, but, paradoxically, because of the lack of nutrients in these foods, the extra calories go hand in hand with nutritional deficiency. The extreme industrialization of food

with no thought for the health of consumers means that overnutrition and malnutrition can occur simultaneously in a population, and sometimes even in the same family. This is truly a tragedy responsible for one of the world's greatest inequalities: one billion people suffer from hunger while two billion are overweight.

Obesity and Cancer

One of the most serious consequences of the obesity epidemic currently sweeping the planet, in both rich and poor countries, is the drastic increase in a number of diseases associated with obesity (Figure 26). Fatty tissue is not an inert mass that just passively stores up extra energy in the form of fat; on the contrary, the cells in this tissue, called adipocytes, are very dynamic and secrete many

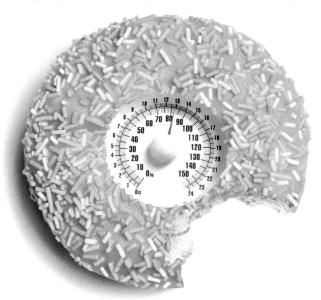

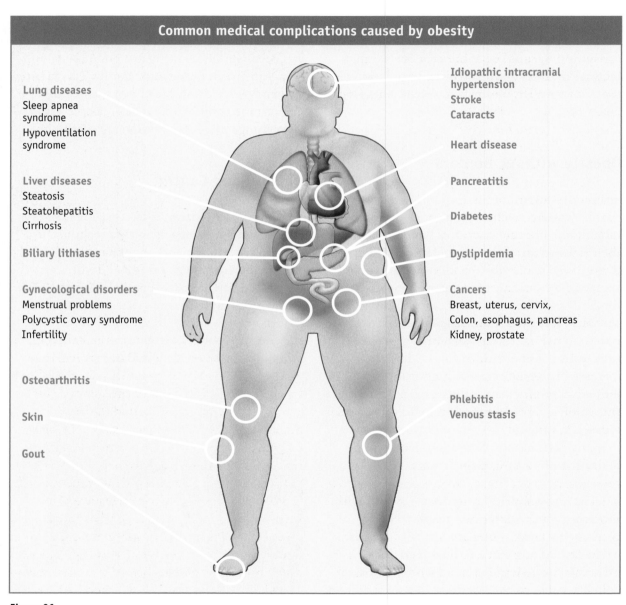

Common medical complications caused by obesity

Lung diseases
Sleep apnea syndrome
Hypoventilation syndrome

Liver diseases
Steatosis
Steatohepatitis
Cirrhosis

Biliary lithiases

Gynecological disorders
Menstrual problems
Polycystic ovary syndrome
Infertility

Osteoarthritis

Skin

Gout

Idiopathic intracranial hypertension
Stroke
Cataracts

Heart disease

Pancreatitis

Diabetes

Dyslipidemia

Cancers
Breast, uterus, cervix,
Colon, esophagus, pancreas
Kidney, prostate

Phlebitis
Venous stasis

Figure 26

hormones, including leptin and adiponectin, which play a very important role in properly regulating metabolism. On the other hand, when adipocytes accumulate too much fat, the stress they undergo disrupts their functioning and creates a climate of low-intensity chronic inflammation that is invisible and undetectable, but that nonetheless upsets the body's overall equilibrium. In obese people, fatty tissue acts just like a magnet to attract the immune system's inflammatory cells, macrophages in particular. The production of inflammatory factors by these cells plays a predominant role in the dramatic rise in the risk of diseases closely related to obesity, like type 2 diabetes and cardiovascular disease.

Several studies indicate that being overweight is also an important cancer risk factor. An increase in BMI is linked to a significant rise in the incidence of this disease and its mortality rate, especially for cancers of the esophagus, endometrium, colon, breast and kidney (Figure 27).

Among the mechanisms at play, the multiplication of certain inflammatory molecules as a result of extra fat creates conditions in which mutations in precancerous cells can occur (see p. 20). In addition, it's interesting to note that several cancers common in obese people occur in organs in the abdominal cavity (endometrium, colon, kidney), perhaps because the excess fat

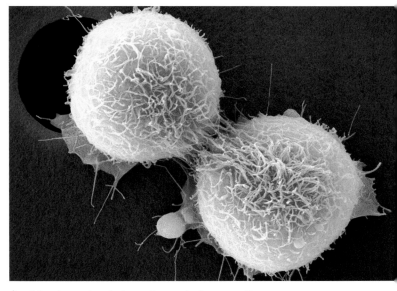

^ Colored scanning electron micrograph of cancer cells.

surrounding these organs creates an environment high in inflammatory molecules in which cancer can thrive. The more extra fat there is, the more favorable the environment. For example, men who have put on 45 pounds (20 kg) in adulthood have a 60% higher risk of developing colon cancer than those who have managed to limit their weight gain to less than 11 pounds (5 kg). The pro-cancer effect of inflammatory molecules is seen even when an overweight person is considered to be in good metabolic health, meaning that he or she does not have any early warning signs of diabetes, high blood pressure or heart disease. Being both obese and in good health is therefore a myth, since overweight

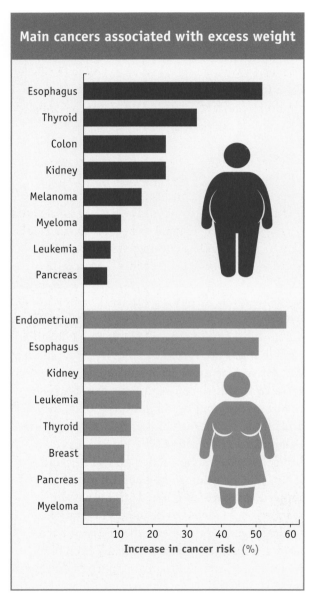

Main cancers associated with excess weight

Esophagus
Thyroid
Colon
Kidney
Melanoma
Myeloma
Leukemia
Pancreas

Endometrium
Esophagus
Kidney
Leukemia
Thyroid
Breast
Pancreas
Myeloma

10   20   30   40   50   60

Increase in cancer risk (%)

Figure 27   Adapted from Khandekar et al., 2011.

people are at higher risk of developing some kinds of cancer than are people of normal weight.

Other factors can also contribute to the increase in cancer risk associated with being overweight. In obese people, steroid hormone levels have been considerably modified, compared with thin people, as a result of the hyperactivity of aromatase, an enzyme that converts androgens into estrogens in fat cells. This surplus estrogen might play an important role in the emergence of cancers that depend on these hormones, like those of the breast, uterus and ovaries. Another of obesity's negative effects is to fundamentally modify sugar metabolism by disrupting the uptake of blood glucose by the organs in response to insulin signaling. Known as insulin resistance, this is associated with an increase in the level of sugar in the bloodstream (hyperglycemia), as well as with a surplus of insulin, secreted in too large a quantity by the pancreas to compensate for its lower level of activity. Over time, the secretory function of the pancreas tapers off, and the decline in insulin results in type 2 diabetes.

Several studies indicate that these disruptions in glucose metabolism could play an important role in the development of certain types of cancer in overweight people. For example, diabetes is associated with an increase of approximately 40% in breast cancer risk, which could explain the alarming increase in this cancer worldwide, given the widespread nature of today's poor food habits. But even in the absence of diabetes, hyperglycemia seems to be enough to increase the risk of cancer, and people with a higher than normal fasting glucose level have twice the risk of dying prematurely from this disease (Figure 28).

Baby Food

In addition to their metabolic effects, industrial foods are sorely lacking in the complex molecules essential for the colon's microbial flora to function properly. Not only are these foods too high in calories, but their energy is too easily absorbed by the intestine and leaves very few substrates to feed the hundreds of billions of bacteria that normally thrive on the complex starches and dietary fiber in food. The starches and fibers in legumes or whole grain bread, for example, are largely fermented in the colon by resident bacteria, which produces beneficial products like short-chain fatty acids that act as anti-inflammatories. This fermentation activity is very important for health, but it currently remains largely untapped, as food is deliberately made to be swallowed and digested quickly, and is thus lacking in these complex molecules. For example, whereas it's estimated that a mouthful of "normal" food has to be chewed about 25 times before being swallowed, the lack of fiber

in industrial foods, combined with their high fat content, which acts as a lubricant, means that only 10 chews on average are needed. Modern industrial food is really "baby food for adults," developed to be ingested with a minimum of effort while providing the body with maximum energy.

Several observations indicate that this kind of food disrupts the equilibrium of the intestinal flora and might contribute to increased risk for some of the cancers associated with obesity. For example, the analysis of stool samples from colon cancer patients shows a decrease in the bacteria that digest dietary

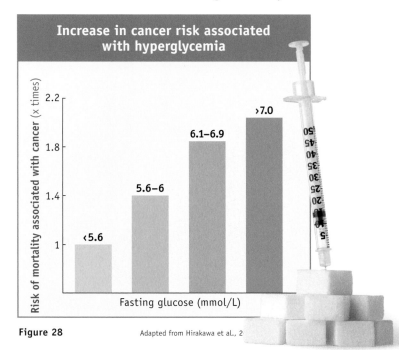

Increase in cancer risk associated with hyperglycemia

Risk of mortality associated with cancer (x times)

‹5.6 — 1
5.6–6 — 1.4
6.1–6.9 — 1.8
›7.0 — ›2.0

Fasting glucose (mmol/L)

Figure 28　　　Adapted from Hirakawa et al., 2

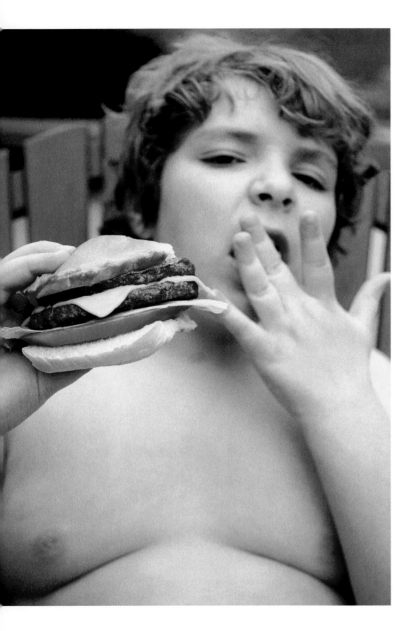

fiber and are known to play a protective role against colorectal cancer, while bacteria whose metabolism generates inflammatory molecules have multiplied significantly. These differences may also contribute to the emergence of liver cancer, since some bacteria commonly found in obese people produce desoxycholic acid, a bile by-product that attacks the DNA of hepatocytes and causes genetic mutations. The composition of the intestinal flora could also play a role in the increase in body weight of obese people, and thus in the ensuing cancer risk, since the bacteria in their intestines are more efficient at extracting energy from food. Industrial livestock breeders have long known that antibiotics speed up weight gain in animals, and some researchers have linked this growth to a disruption in the intestinal flora that would favor bacteria with a "higher energy output." Whether or not this is the case, these changes in bacterial flora are not irreversible, and by simply incorporating plenty of plant foods into our diet we can re-establish the levels of useful bacteria and enjoy their positive effect on health.

21st Century Tobacco

The chronic exposure of the population to cheap foods, overloaded with sugar and fat and promoted by never-ending, flashy advertising campaigns, is mainly to blame for the explosion in obesity that is currently ravaging the planet. This way of eating is disastrous for health; our metabolism has evolved to function optimally in conditions of food scarcity and is completely unsuited to this overabundance of food energy. The metabolic disorders and chronic inflammation caused by too much weight thus create ideal conditions for the emergence of several diseases, including cancer. Furthermore, owing to the globalization of obesity, we can see in real time the disastrous consequences of current dietary habits for cancer risk, with more than 22 million new cases of cancer a year expected to occur in developing countries. Already dealing with cancers related to infections (liver, stomach and cervical cancer), these countries are now also faced with cancers they very seldom used to see, like breast and colon cancer, a result of the consumption of industrialized food products exported by rich countries, as well as obesity and lack of exercise.

As with tobacco dependence, obesity is essentially the unfortunate outcome of an ideology in which the financial interests of a number of companies with no consideration for consumers' well-being take precedence. Furthermore, the penetration of emerging markets by industrial food products occurs in tandem with an increase in smoking, which suggests

similar marketing strategies. This parallel between the junk food and tobacco industries is striking when we examine the strategies used by food giants to justify their marketing practices (Figure 29). In both cases, the act of consuming a product is an individual choice, and it's thus consumers' responsibility to avoid the excesses that might put their health in danger.

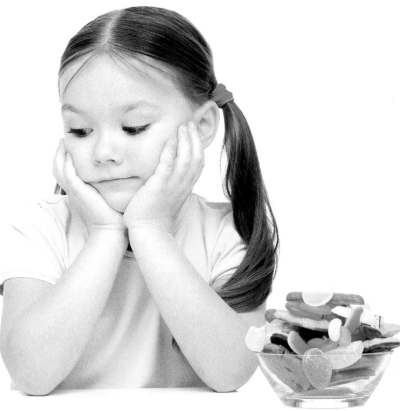

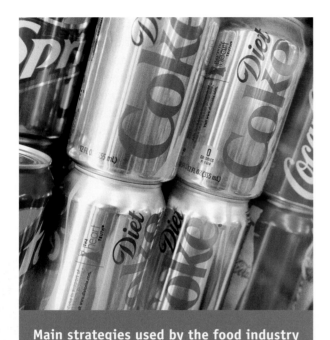

Main strategies used by the food industry to justify marketing its products

- Invoke personal responsibility as the cause of widespread poor diet.
- Maintain that increased government regulation would be an attack on individual liberties.
- Denigrate critics by using extremist language.
- Retaliate against unfavorable studies by undermining them.
- Put the spotlight on physical activity rather than diet.
- Declare that foods are neither good nor bad in themselves.

Figure 29

Other much more insidious and unfortunately often repeated arguments the industry uses are that foods are neither good nor bad and that only consuming too much is harmful. Yet the current obesity epidemic could never have occurred if there were no bad foods! Studies clearly show that regularly consuming carbonated beverages or fast-food meals, even when amounts are not excessive, is associated with a marked increase in the risk of obesity and diseases stemming from it, even in young people. It is therefore the increasing number of these products and changes in food habits that are the real problem and the cause of the deterioration in health observed even in regions formerly taken as dietary reference points (Okinawa and Crete). We have to be critical of this industry and realize that the highly processed foods they offer are bad for our health, quite simply because the long-term risks of consuming them outweigh their short-term benefits. The example of cigarettes shows that a substance that is nontoxic in the short term can become toxic in the longer term, given regular consumption. We must not repeat the error made with tobacco by waiting until the damage caused by obesity reaches excessive proportions before taking action. Faced with this industry, consumers must look after themselves, and public health authorities must adopt appropriate measures to protect society's most vulnerable, who are especially targeted by such irresponsible commercial practices.

We can justly congratulate ourselves on the significant decline in smoking in recent decades, but we must be aware that the increase in obesity could on its own wipe out the benefits of the decrease in the number of smokers. The situation is made even more worrying by the fact that an increasing number of children are overweight or obese. In the United States, for example, childhood obesity has almost quadrupled in 30 years; 15% of children from 6 to 11 years of age were obese in 2000. The vast majority of these children will still be obese in adulthood and will, as a result, be at high risk of developing several types of cancer related to obesity. The fight against obesity thus requires very rapid intervention, starting in early childhood, especially since the risk of obesity takes hold very early on — half of children and teenagers who become obese are already overweight when they start kindergarten.

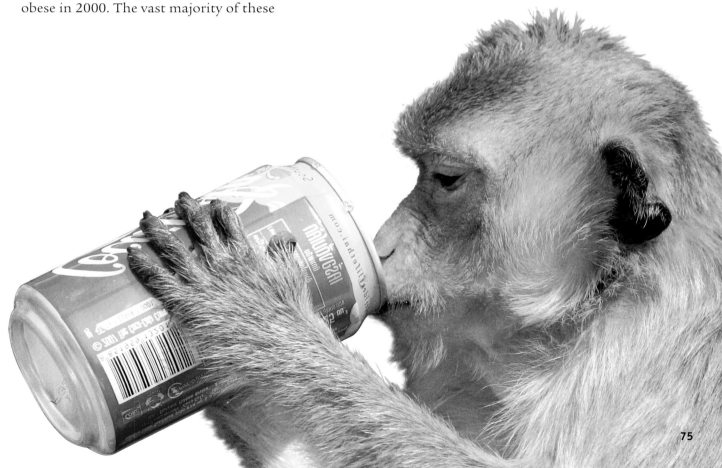

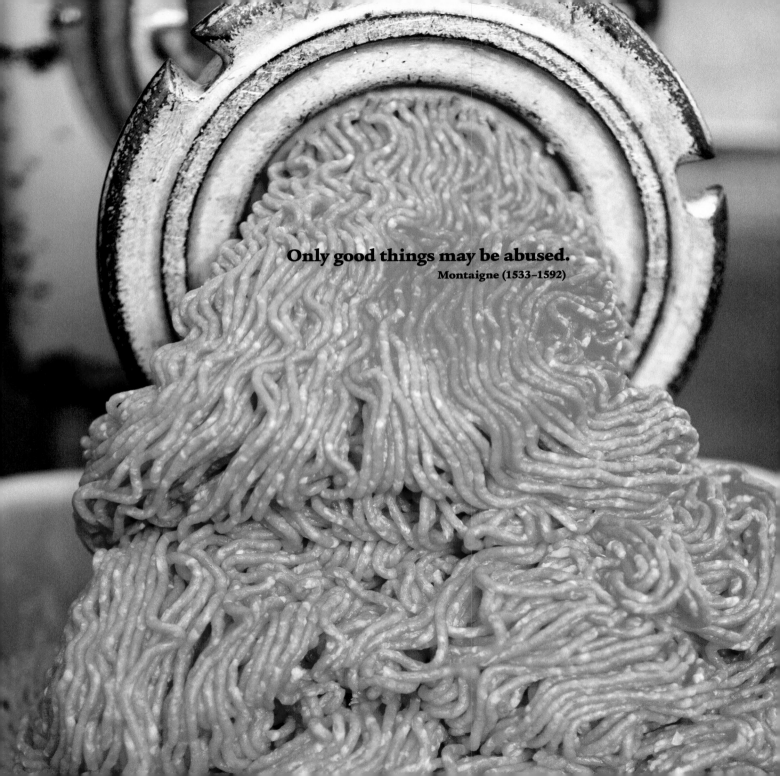

Only good things may be abused.

Montaigne (1533–1592)

Chapter 4

Meat: When Cancer Sees Red

Recommendation

Limit the consumption of red meat (beef, lamb, pork) to approximately 1 pound (500 g) per week, replacing it with meals based on fish, eggs or vegetable proteins.

Source: World Cancer Research Fund International

In French, the word for meat — *viande* — derived from the Latin *vivenda* ("what is used for life"), long referred to solid food in general, whether bread, vegetables, nuts or more elaborate dishes based on animal flesh or fish. For example, during the ceremony that surrounded every one of Louis the XIV's dinners at Versailles, when "Messieurs, à la viande du roi" was announced, it wasn't so much the animal flesh that was referred to, as the "vital" substance of the meal as a whole, indispensable to the Sun King's life. It was only later that the word viande would be exclusively used to refer to pigs, cattle, fowl and other edible animals, a shift in meaning that likely reflected an innate attraction to these foods, as well as their pervasiveness in the human diet.

A number of social, cultural and economic factors can be cited to explain the predominance of meat, but the main reason is a very simple one: most people love meat quite simply because meat tastes good! Although raw meat holds very little culinary interest, its cooking unleashes a very complex chain of chemical reactions that create thousands of extraordinarily aromatic molecules, ranging from 2-methyl-3-furanthiol

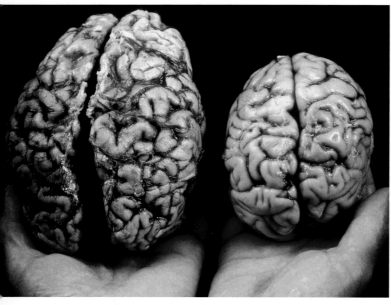

^ On the left, a human brain, and on the right, the brain of a gorilla.

and inosinate, two molecules detected by receptors in the tongue's taste buds. These receptors are specialized in detecting the taste of umami (from the Japanese umai, "delicious," and mi, "taste"), signaling to the brain the presence of a protein-rich food, and in so doing activating the brain's pleasure and reward centers, which make meat dishes so appealing. And it can be hard to resist them — the amniotic fluid surrounding a fetus is rich in glutamate, meaning that right from the beginning of our lives, our pleasure center has been stimulated by exposure to this substance

From Herbivore to Omnivore

Human beings' attraction to meat is nothing new. Approximately 3 million years ago, our distant ancestor *Homo habilis* abandoned the traditional diet of the great apes, almost exclusively based on plants, and began to add to it meat from the remains of carcasses left behind by predators, in so doing acquiring a taste for animal flesh and becoming a hunter. This was a dangerous exercise, to say the least, for being small in size — 3 feet 11 inches (1.2 m) and 88 pounds (40 kg) — not very fast, and lacking claws and sharp teeth, *Homo habilis* had none of the traits of a hunter, let alone a predator! But this change would have extraordinary consequences for our subsequent evolution. Since it is very high in calories and

to 3-mercapto-2-pentanone, and including hundreds of volatile substances produced by the reaction between meat's sugars and proteins. Some of these molecules give off an aroma that is reminiscent of fruits, and others, of mushrooms or nuts, but collectively they are combined by our brain to produce a new aroma, one that is unknown in nature and only exists because of cooking: the incomparable aroma produced by cooking a piece of meat.

And that's not all! In addition to its unique aroma, cooking meat also releases glutamate

78

Nourishing the Brain

Even though the human brain makes up just 2% of body weight, it alone consumes 20% of the entire energy of the resting organism. Maintaining an alert brain thus requires a considerable energy intake of about 6 calories per billion neurons. For the human brain's phenomenal development during evolution to occur, our distant ancestors therefore had to increase their caloric intake by about 700 calories a day.

There is no doubt that it would have been very difficult to meet this kind of demand by retaining the great apes' herbivorous diet; a primitive human being eating only plant foods located in the immediate vicinity would have had to spend more than 9 hours a day eating to get these extra calories, which was of course impossible, given the time needed to find and gather so much food.

Eating meat made it possible to resolve this energy problem and acted as a catalyst for the evolution of the human brain. On the one hand, since it was high in calories and contained a large quantity of essential vitamins and minerals, meat was able to meet the basic energy needs required for increased brain functioning. But in addition, and even more importantly, this increased intelligence was then used to make

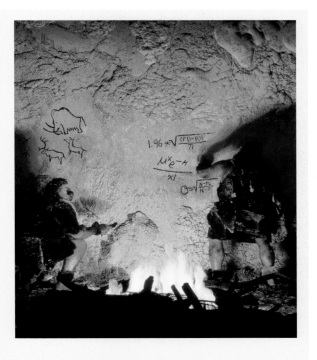

tools that made it easier to obtain meat and foods that were very high in energy and that had formerly been inaccessible, like bone marrow or brains, two major sources of the polyunsaturated fat necessary for neuronal development. Having become more intelligent, humans were able to domesticate fire and invent cooking, making food easier to digest and, as a result, increasing calorie and essential nutrient intake. A better diet was associated with earlier weaning of children and thus with a higher number of births per woman, which meant that the human population could increase more rapidly.

essential nutrients, meat was able to provide the extra energy needed for brain development, thus triggering an amplification loop conducive to the phenomenal development of our species' brain capacity (see box p. 79). Their rash behavior turned these simple, vulnerable gatherers into fearsome predators, able to use their intelligence to obtain a precious energy source in the form of meat. All the same, these new food habits did not turn us into carnivores! We enjoy and digest meat, of course, but we have neither the anatomy (teeth, jaws, stomach) nor the physiology (uric acid metabolism) of animals that get their essential food supply from animal flesh. We are actually omnivores biologically designed to eat mainly plant-based foods, but culturally adapted to diversify and supplement this diet by incorporating into it various foods from animal sources.

The Red and the White

Meat of the kind we eat today is very different from the wild game of the prehistoric era and is the fruit of the considerable efforts early civilizations put into domesticating wild animals. Whether it was the sheep, goats or cattle of southeastern Turkey 10,000 years ago, the pigs of Turkey and Asia 8,000 years ago or the chickens of Southeast Asia in the same period — all these animals made it possible for humans to be able to count on a regular supply of meat, despite a more sedentary way of life. It's absolutely remarkable that, 10,000 years later, these same animals remain the mainstays of the human diet, with chicken, beef and pork alone making up 90% of all the meat eaten every year in Canada (Figure 30).

All of this meat, whether it comes from cattle, sheep, pigs or fowl, is muscle of similar structure, made up of muscle fibers, adipose tissue (fat) and connective tissue (collagen). There are, however, significant differences in the proportions of these various components, especially in their fat content, which can range from barely 1% in fowl to more than

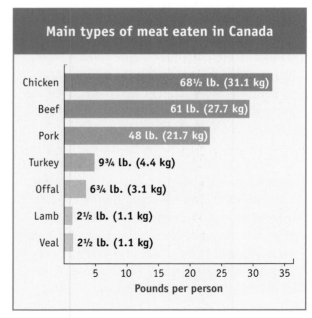

Main types of meat eaten in Canada

Meat	Pounds per person
Chicken	68½ lb. (31.1 kg)
Beef	61 lb. (27.7 kg)
Pork	48 lb. (21.7 kg)
Turkey	9¾ lb. (4.4 kg)
Offal	6¾ lb. (3.1 kg)
Lamb	2½ lb. (1.1 kg)
Veal	2½ lb. (1.1 kg)

Figure 30 Adapted from Robitaille, 2012.

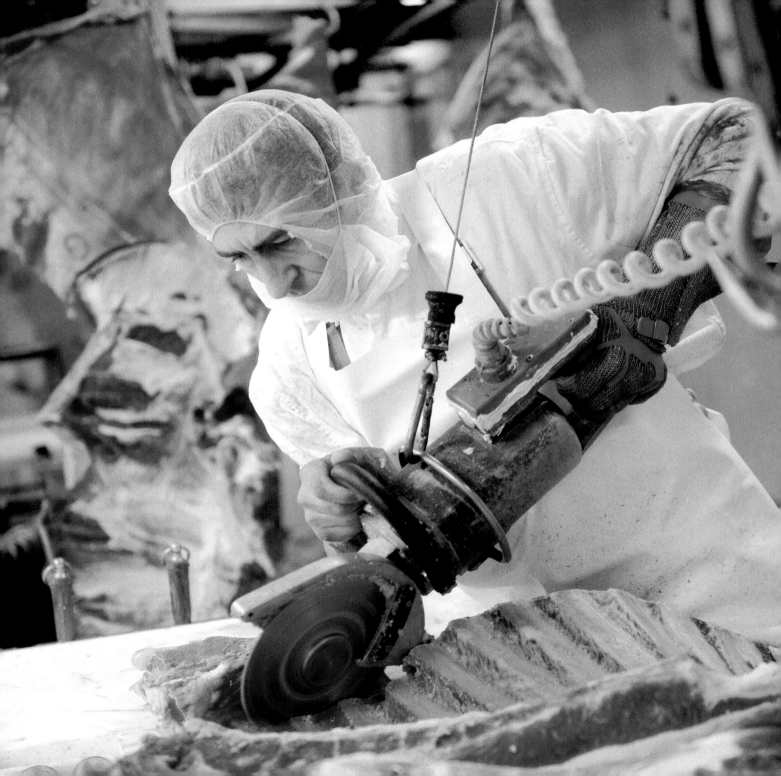

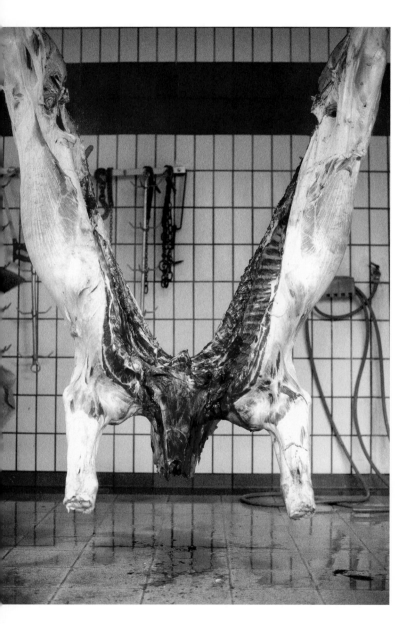

30% in beef, depending on the cut. This fat content is in large part responsible for the very distinct flavors of these meats, especially when it is located between the muscle fibers (the "marbling" in beef, for example, so highly prized by beef lovers, is in fact intramuscular fat). However, the most visible difference between these types of meat is their color: beef and pork, as well as lamb and horse, are what are called red meats, whereas fowl like chicken and turkey are white meats. But what causes these differences in color? What may appear at first glance to be an insignificant question is, on the contrary, of great importance in understanding the different effects of meat on health.

Red meat

Contrary to what many people think, meat is not red because it contains blood. Its color actually comes from its high myoglobin content. Myoglobin is a protein that can bind oxygen by interacting with a heme group, a structure that contains an atom of iron. This heme iron enables myoglobin to store oxygen in the muscles and thus to sustain the intense metabolic activity needed for muscular contraction. Muscles that are used for long periods, like those involved in maintaining balance or walking, need more oxygen to function and as a result have a higher myoglobin content (1–2% in cattle,

0.2% in pigs). In wild animals (bison, moose), which are much more active, the quantity of myoglobin can even reach such high levels that the meat sometimes looks black.

It is the changes in this interaction of myoglobin with oxygen that cause the variations in color that occur during the storage or cooking of red meat. For example, when the temperature reaches approximately 140°F (60°C), the iron in the myoglobin loses an electron (we then say it has oxidized) and from then on can no longer capture oxygen, which causes the brownish color typical of cooked meat.

The color of meat can also be chemically modified. In some countries, a small amount of carbon monoxide (CO) is sometimes added to meat, which prevents myoglobin from oxidizing and gives a more appealing red color to packaged meats. However, the meat's brilliant red color can last even after the meat has gone bad, posing an increased risk of food poisoning. Another example of artificial coloring is "pink slime," an industrial paste made from a mixture of shredded beef trimmings treated with ammonia to eliminate bacteria. These alkaline conditions give the meat a very unappetizing pink color, which does not, however, keep the United States from authorizing its commercial use as a filling agent for ground beef or processed meats, like cold cuts.

Processed meats

The preparation of meat in the form of processed meat products goes back to ancient times, this technique having been used to increase the length of time meat could be preserved before refrigeration was invented. This is because meat's nutritional value does not just appeal to human beings; micro-organisms also love it and can quickly make it unfit for eating. The Greeks and Romans, for example, stuffed the viscera or stomachs of animals with blood or pieces of finely chopped meat, to which they added salt, spices and aromatics as preserving agents. The use of large amounts of salt is especially important, as salt partially dehydrates the meat, thus reducing the humidity that fosters the proliferation of pathogens. In fact, the word "sausage" comes from the Latin *salsus*, meaning salty.

The first specialty butchers, including the Greek chef Aphtonite, whom some claim was the inventor of blood sausage, did not know that the salt they were using contained traces of saltpeter (potassium nitrate).

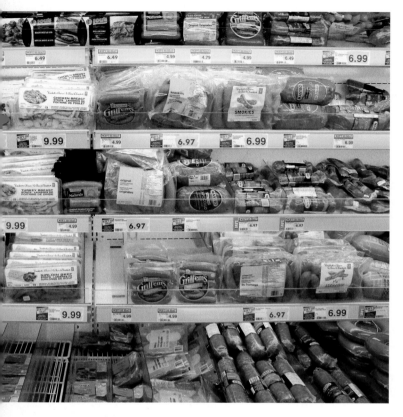

White meat

White meat is made up of so-called "fast" muscle fibers, which are adapted so that the organism can exert itself for a short period of time without using oxygen. These muscles therefore have no myoglobin, or very little, and instead derive their energy from glycogen, a glucose polymer that acts as a reservoir for sugar as a "fuel" required for muscle contraction. Fowl such as chicken or turkey fly very little and are adapted to make sudden but short movements with their wings; as a result, their chest muscles are almost entirely lacking in myoglobin. On the other hand, these animals walk a lot, and their thighs need more oxygen to maintain the pace — hence their higher myoglobin levels and darker color (brown) of these muscles.

Carnivores at Risk

This was a lucky accident, as these nitrates are powerful antibacterial agents, and this property definitely saved a good many people from potentially deadly poisonings, like those caused by the lethal *Clostridium botulinum* (botulism). Another advantage of nitrates is that they decompose into nitrites, and then into nitrous oxide (NO), a gas that can attach itself to myoglobin, turning meat a pinkish color that can last for several weeks.

Whereas meat was once a luxury product, sometimes very expensive and as such reserved for important occasions, it's now common in the modern diet as a result of its wide availability and lower cost, both made possible by large-scale industrialization of agriculture. With the notable exception of India, where 40% of the population does not eat animals at all, or seldom, for religious reasons, meat consumption has literally exploded in most

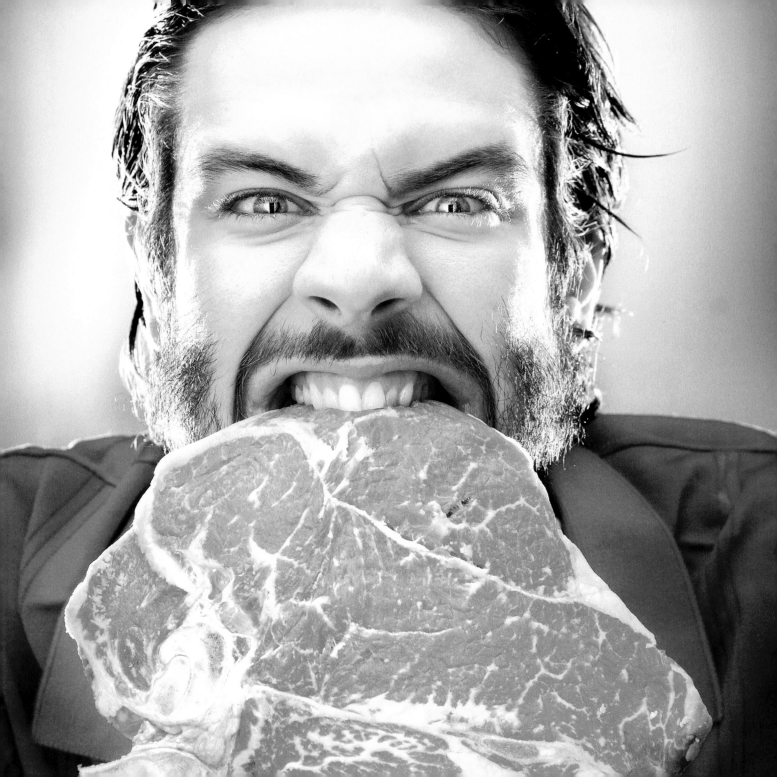

parts of the world. For example, developing countries in the Middle East or eastern Asia, whose people traditionally ate little meat, have doubled and even in some cases quintupled their meat consumption, a trend that is likely to continue in the coming years. Industrialized countries, however, remain the undisputed champions in this field, with each person eating on average twice as much meat as people in the rest of the world.

It has long been known that a diet high in red meat and low in plant foods combined with too much body weight and a highly sedentary lifestyle is associated with a higher incidence of colorectal cancer. The impact of this way of life is striking, with the industrialized countries like those of North America and Europe having a colon cancer rate five to 30 times higher than that of India and certain countries in the Middle East and Africa (Figure 31).

Japan offers a striking example of the speed with which the industrialization of a society can impact cancer risk. Heirs to a long dietary tradition based on the plentiful consumption

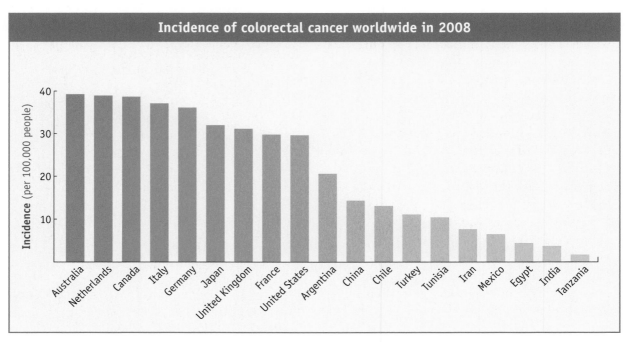

Figure 31

Adapted from Globocan, 2008.

of seafood and legumes like soy, the Japanese have radically changed their diet since the end of World War II, with an astonishing jump (700%) in their meat consumption, especially red meat, and an increase in the number of overweight people. The Japanese had one of the lowest incidences of colorectal cancer in the world just 30 years ago; these major changes in their lifestyle have resulted in a 400% increase in the incidence of this cancer, with its current rate now similar to that of several countries in Europe and the Americas. This increase is seen very early on, by the time people are in their late thirties, which suggests that exposure to the western way of life causes the rapid formation of precancerous lesions and speeds up their development dramatically (Figure 32).

Red meat and processed meat are often singled out to explain the high incidence of colorectal cancer in industrialized countries. Several studies show that people who eat a lot of these kinds of meat see their risk of getting this cancer rise by approximately 30% in comparison with those who eat only very small amounts. Every 1¾ ounce (50 g) daily serving of red meat or processed meat increases this risk by about 10%, with people who eat more than 4¼ ounces (120 g) per day at highest risk (Figure 33). This effect occurs only in the case of red meat; consuming chicken or fish has no impact on cancer risk.

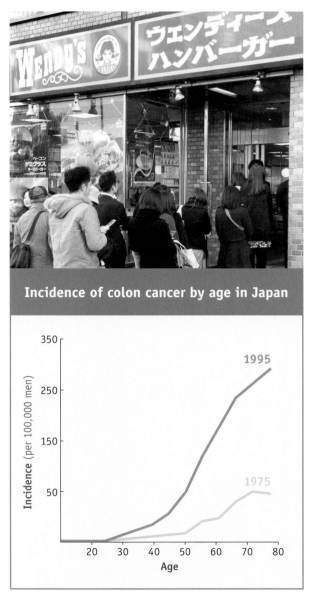

Incidence of colon cancer by age in Japan

Figure 32   Adapted from Kuriki and Tajima, 2006.

The harmful effect of red meat on colorectal cancer risk has repercussions for life expectancy. A huge study of half a million people showed that eating red meat and meat products was associated with a linear increase in mortality risk, with people who eat 5½ ounces (160 g) per day having a 50% higher risk of dying prematurely (Figure 34). Subsequent analyses suggest that this negative effect is particularly due to processed meats (bacon, sausages, salami, ham), responsible for an increase of 20 to 40% in mortality in those who consume the largest amounts, whereas people who eat the most fresh red meat daily (beef, pork, lamb) see their risk of premature death increase by 13% in comparison with those who eat little or none.

Carcinogen Production

The negative impact on health of eating an excessive amount of red meat is a reflection of its high caloric density as well as the major biochemical changes it undergoes during cooking or preserving. First of all, it cannot be denied that red meat's high calorie content, so important for our evolution, is not adapted to the current overabundance of food, with the result that people who eat a lot of meat have a higher risk of being overweight or obese. In addition, several studies have shown that increased consumption of red meat is

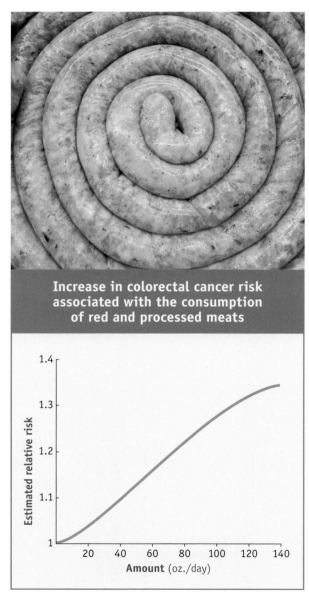

Increase in colorectal cancer risk associated with the consumption of red and processed meats

Figure 33

Adapted from Chan et al., 2011.

associated with a higher risk of type 2 diabetes, a disease closely tied to being overweight. Since obesity is a major risk factor for several cancers (see Chapter 3), especially colon cancer, the calorie surplus caused by eating too much red meat can therefore certainly contribute to the increase in this cancer.

Several other factors are suspected to play a role in the proliferation of cancers in people who eat large amounts of red meat and processed meat products. The heme iron content of these foods, for example, creates free radicals and promotes the formation of N-nitroso compounds, which have the dangerous property of being able to attach themselves randomly to our genetic material and introduce mutations into our DNA. Since processed meat products are major sources of these carcinogenic compounds and also contain nitrites that can be changed into nitrosamines, these molecules may contribute to the negative effects of these prepared meats in several parts of the world.

Cooking might also reinforce the negative effects of red meat on health. At high temperatures (>400°F or 200°C), creatine

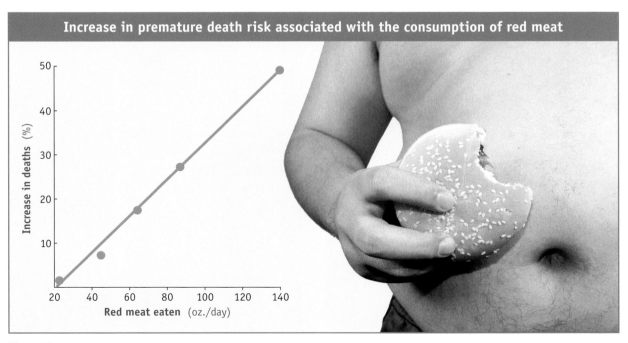

Increase in premature death risk associated with the consumption of red meat

Red meat eaten (oz./day)

Increase in deaths (%)

Figure 34

Adapted from Sinha et al., 2009.

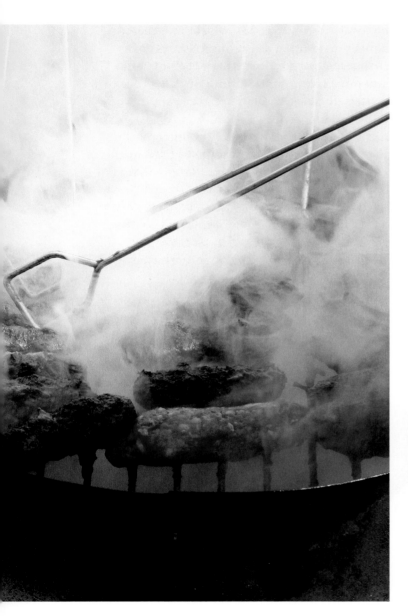

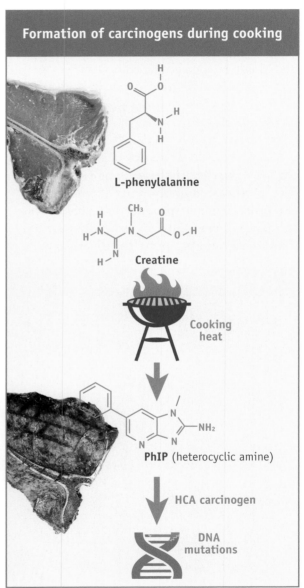

Figure 35

found in large amounts in the muscle cells combines chemically with the amino acids in proteins to form heterocyclic amines (HCAs) that also have the ability to attach themselves to our DNA and trigger the development of a cancer (Figure 35).

These complex molecules are easy to see: the more charred the meat, the higher the HCA content. Beef, for example, has a low level of HCA when cooked for less time (medium), but in meat that is well done, the quantity of carcinogens triples, and it can reach very high amounts in some preparations like bacon (Figure 36). Fifteen or so of these carcinogenic molecules have been identified in meat cooked at high temperature, and some studies have shown that high consumption of charred meat is associated with an increase in risk for colon, pancreatic and prostate cancer.

However, it's very easy to eliminate nearly all of these molecules by marinating meat in virgin olive oil with garlic and lemon juice (Figure 37) or herbs like thyme or rosemary. These marinades also make it possible to reduce by 70% the production of malonaldehyde, a by-product of animal fat that increases the risk of heart disease. Asian-style marinades, containing for example teriyaki sauce or

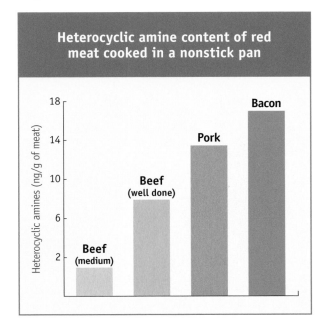

Heterocyclic amine content of red meat cooked in a nonstick pan

Heterocyclic amines (ng/g of meat)

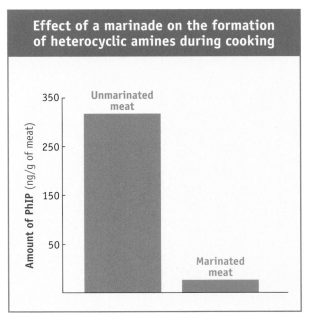

Effect of a marinade on the formation of heterocyclic amines during cooking

Amount of PhIP (ng/g of meat)

Figure 36   Adapted from Puangsombat et al., 2012.   **Figure 37**   Adapted from Salmon et al., 1997.

turmeric, also decrease by a third the production of heterocyclic amines, whereas commercial barbecue sauces triple the production of these carcinogens. Even busy people can cut the formation of heterocyclic amines approximately in half simply by adding turmeric (0.2%) or related spices (krachai, galangal) to ground beef before cooking (Figure 38). The possibilities are endless and confirm the ancestral knowledge of Caribbean culinary traditions, which always used meat marinated with spices and aromatics for *barbacòa,* the ancestor of today's barbecue.

Today's Meat

The boom in red meat production, made possible by large-scale agricultural industrialization, has led to major changes in the composition of meat. Although beef cattle are ruminants that normally eat grasses like clover and alfalfa, these animals are now fattened with corn and soy to speed up their growth and get them to slaughter sooner. These changes to the bovine diet have major repercussions for the composition of the meat,

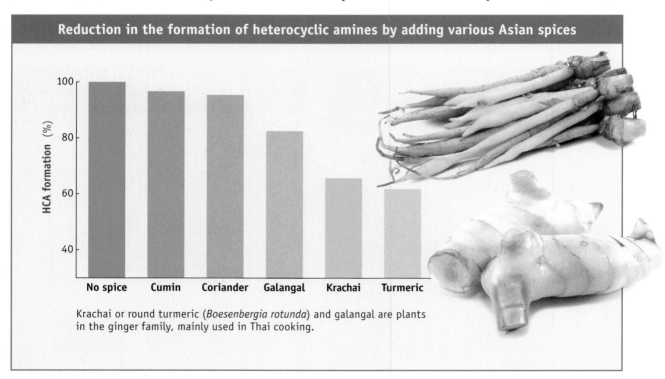

Reduction in the formation of heterocyclic amines by adding various Asian spices

HCA formation (%)

No spice · Cumin · Coriander · Galangal · Krachai · Turmeric

Krachai or round turmeric (*Boesenbergia rotunda*) and galangal are plants in the ginger family, mainly used in Thai cooking.

Figure 38

Adapted from Puangsombat et al., 2011.

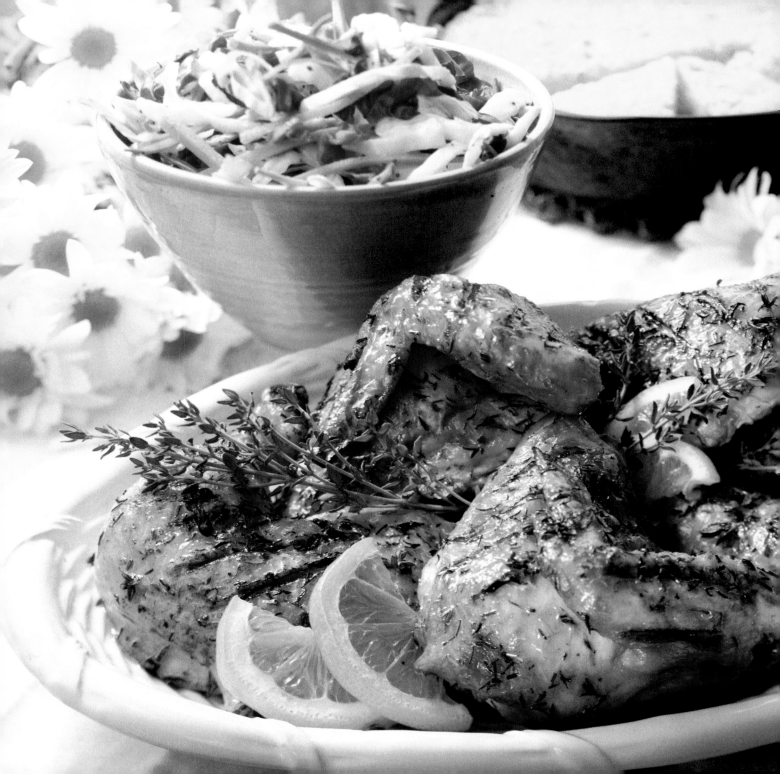

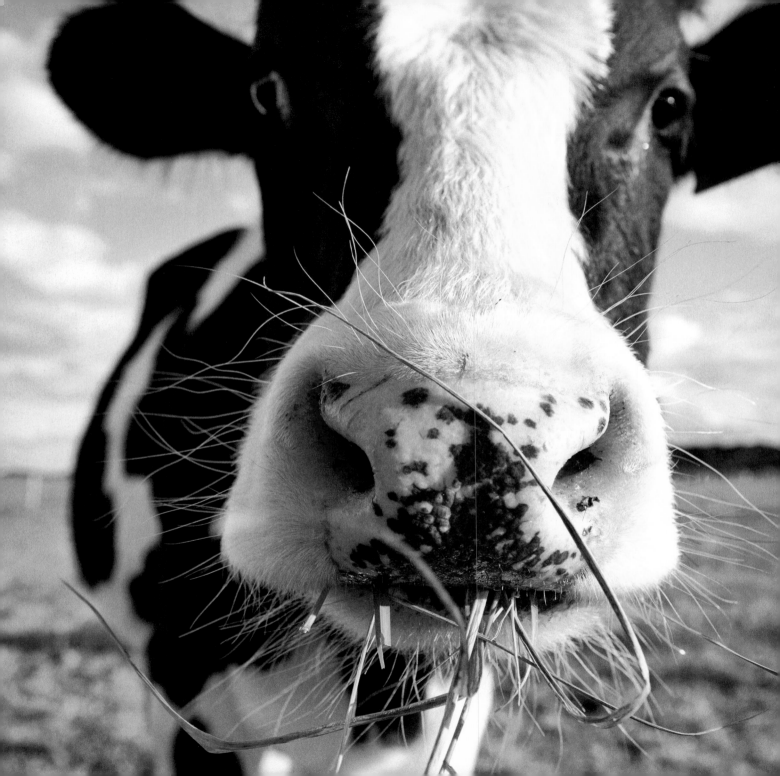

since corn is a source of starch and therefore of sugar, and this sugar is converted into fat by the animal. Consequently, meat from cattle fed in this way has roughly twice as much fat as meat from exclusively grass-fed animals, with this fat accumulating right inside the muscles. The marbling in most cuts of beef now on the market therefore indicates an animal whose growth was sped up artificially by feeding it too much sugar.

This kind of diet also has a major influence on meat's essential pro-inflammatory omega-6 and anti-inflammatory omega-3 fats. Since corn has no omega-3, animals fed this grain have one- third as much anti-inflammatory fat in their meat as grass-fed animals (Figure 39). The opposite is true for omega-6 fats, as the meat of cattle fed with corn contains twice as much of these inflammatory fats. The consequences of this change in bovine diet are therefore huge, with today's meat now having an omega-6/omega-3 ratio of about 13, compared with a ratio of 2 for the meat of animals fed in the traditional way. This is a critical difference, as the western diet contains 10 to 30 times more omega-6 fats than omega-3 fats, contributing to the creation inside the body of an inflammatory environment that can foster the onset of a number of chronic diseases. With regard to cancer, it's also interesting to note that Argentina, where eating meat from pasture-raised — and thus grass-fed — cattle is

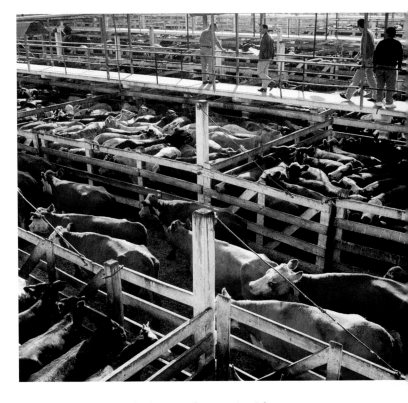

part of the national identity, has an incidence of colorectal cancer that is nearly half that of Canada, despite beef consumption that is twice as high (128 pounds or 58 kg/person, compared with 59½ pounds or 27 kg). It's often said that we are what we eat, which is no doubt true, but we are also what is eaten by what we eat, and it's very likely that the extreme industrialization of livestock farming related to red meat production contributes to the negative effects associated with eating too much of these foods.

There are therefore several reasons for the harmful effects of overconsumption of red meat and processed meats on health, ranging from the high calorie content of these foods, to the production of cancer-causing compounds when they are cooked or preserved, to their abnormally low anti-inflammatory omega-3 fatty acid content. It must be remembered as well that studies have shown that big meat-eaters usually eat fewer plant foods, thus depriving themselves of precious allies in preventing cancer. For example, studies have shown that green vegetables like spinach can reverse the damage caused by the heme iron or

HCAs in meat by reducing the oncogenic impact of these toxic molecules.

Significant Collateral Damage

More than 53 billion animals are killed every year for human consumption, and it goes without saying that livestock farming has enormous repercussions for the environment. Greenhouse gases, the large-scale use of arable land and water to produce grains destined for animal feed, and the confinement of animals in restricted spaces are all consequences of

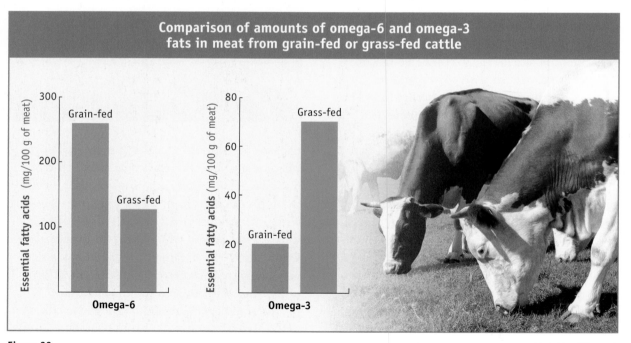

Figure 39

Adapted from Miller, 1986.

intensive livestock farming that can in the medium and long term cause major upheavals in the planetary ecosystem.

The massive use of antibiotics is another kind of collateral damage from large-scale livestock farming that could have serious consequences for human health. During the 1940s, it was noticed that animals given antibiotics grew faster and reached a larger size, which made it possible to reduce production costs and sell meat at more affordable prices. Initially used as medicines for sick animals, antibiotics have now become an integral part of livestock farming, and are given even to healthy animals. In the United States, it's estimated that approximately 1/100 ounce (300 mg) of antibiotics are used to produce each 2¼ pounds (1 kg) of meat and eggs, and that nearly 80% of all the antibiotics used in that country are consumed by livestock. It's also disturbing to realize that larger amounts of antibiotics are given to healthy animals than are used to treat sick people (Figure 40).

Bacteria have an unequalled ability to adapt to adversity. As a result, even though most bacteria are eliminated through the use of antibiotics, the continual use of these drugs exerts evolutionary pressure that forces some bacteria to acquire the ability to resist them. The inappropriate and excessive use of antibiotics thus creates conditions that foster

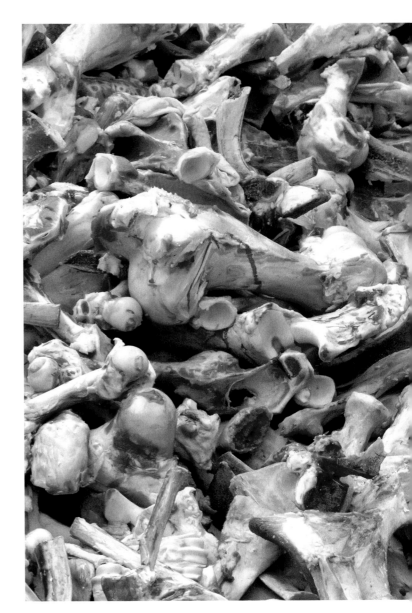

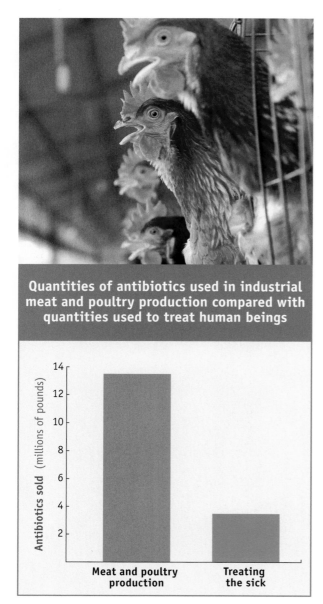

Quantities of antibiotics used in industrial meat and poultry production compared with quantities used to treat human beings

Figure 40   Adapted from www.pewhealth.org, 2013.

the emergence of new strains of resistant bacteria in animals, and this resistance can subsequently be transmitted to bacteria that infect human beings.

This is an alarming situation that we cannot allow ourselves to ignore. It was the discovery of penicillin, followed by a hundred other new antibiotics, that was mainly responsible for the dramatic increase in life expectancy in the 20th century. Before these discoveries, people who contracted infectious diseases like tuberculosis, pneumonia or severe diarrhea often died prematurely, owing to the ineffectiveness of existing treatments. Antibiotics are, in this regard, one of the greatest achievements in the history of science, enabling us to combat serious infections successfully and save countless lives.

Fewer and fewer new antibiotics are being discovered and produced by the pharmaceutical industry, and unless these drugs are used more judiciously and restricted to treating sick animals, we will sooner or later be faced with bacterial diseases against which our current therapeutic arsenal will be powerless. Cases of antibiotic-resistant tuberculosis have exploded in recent years, killing 170,000 people in 2012, and the American Centers for Disease Control and Prevention have identified 17 micro-organisms resistant to antibiotics that cause the deaths of 23,000 people annually.

Replace It With What?

Most public health agencies recommend two to three daily servings of meat and meat substitutes for an adult, which equals about 5½–8½ ounces (160–240 g) of protein. It's somewhat unfair to refer to such healthy and high-quality foods as legumes, nuts and eggs as "substitutes," as they are sources of high-quality proteins every bit as good as those in meat. And these alternatives can literally save lives. When red meat is replaced by other protein sources, whether fish, fowl, nuts or legumes, the increase in the risk of premature mortality associated with red meat is sharply reduced, dropping from 20% to 7%. And let's not forget fatty fish like mackerel, sardines and salmon, major sources of long-chain omega-3 fatty acids, and eicosapentaenoic (EPA) and docosahexaenoic acid (DHA), which can help maintain an anti-inflammatory anticancer environment in the tissues.

Meat's good taste must not make us forget that the amount of animal flesh now commonly consumed in our society far exceeds the recommended amounts, and that it's important to diversify sources of dietary protein. Including plant foods in the diet is in this respect especially important, since people who eat a lot of protein from animal sources (meat, dairy products) have four times the risk of dying from the effects of cancer compared with those who mainly eat proteins from plant sources.

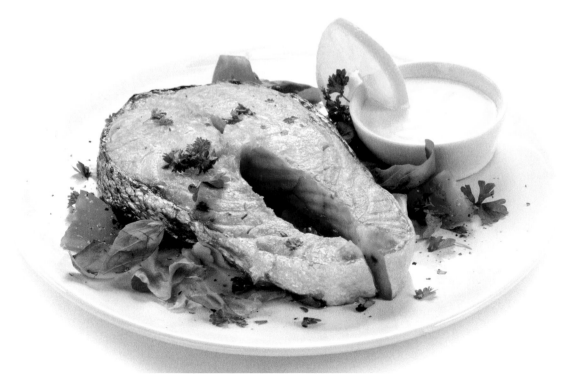

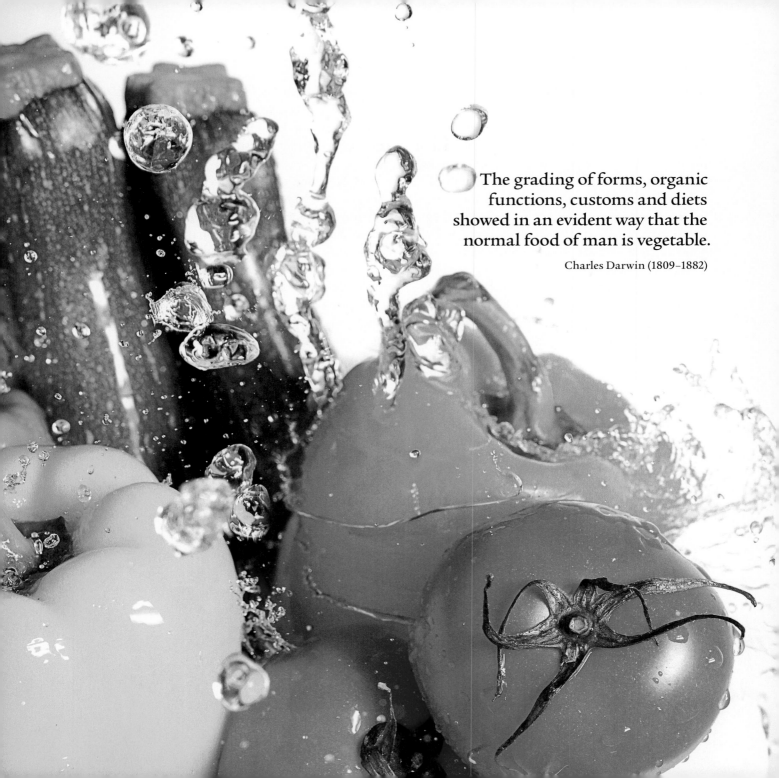

The grading of forms, organic functions, customs and diets showed in an evident way that the normal food of man is vegetable.

Charles Darwin (1809–1882)

Chapter 5

Plants Show Cancer Their True Colors!

Recommendation

Eat more of a variety of fruits, vegetables and legumes, as well as foods based on whole grains. These foods should make up two-thirds of a meal.

Source: World Cancer Research Fund International

The negative impact of the modern industrial diet on the health of both the population and the planet is an alarm signal that we are on the wrong track and that eating is about more than satisfying our hunger with foods overloaded with calories, without considering their harmful effects on our well-being and that of the world around us. The purpose of eating is not just to meet our energy needs; eating is the only way to provide our body with a whole range of elements indispensable to the functioning of our cells and our body's overall equilibrium.

One reason why eating too many highly processed industrial products is so harmful is that these foods make up a larger and larger proportion of our daily meals (up to 60% of all the calories consumed by people in some industrialized societies), to the detriment of foods that are major sources of protective elements key to maintaining good health, especially fruits and vegetables. Just like consuming too many calories, not eating enough plant products is an aspect of the modern diet that contributes to the development of all chronic diseases, including cancer.

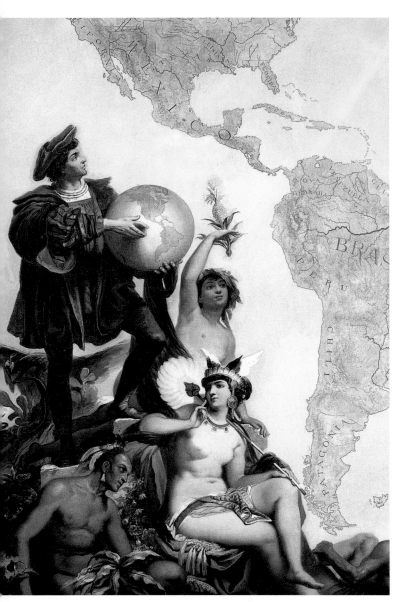

^ "Christopher Columbus and the discovery of America," detail from *Allegory of the Dominions of Charles V*, by Cesare Dell'Acqua (1821–1905).

Plant Globalization

The special relationship between human beings and plant-based foods goes back a very long way. From prehistoric hunter-gatherers to the first explorers who crisscrossed the globe looking for unknown lands, the discovery of new edible plants has always been one of the main concerns of our species, both to ensure survival and to experience a wider range of culinary choices. The identification of nearly 7,000 plants useful for food among the some 500,000 plant species that exist on earth attests to the efforts devoted to this undertaking, especially since each civilization has managed to identify in its own environment those plants containing large amounts of substances beneficial to health. Furthermore, it was because of this curiosity and desire for novelty that the discovery of America by Christopher Columbus was accompanied by the first real "globalization" of food, an exchange of plants that led Italians to begin using the South American tomato to enhance their cooking, helped Indians prepare even spicier curries using Mexican chilies, and made the Peruvian potato indispensable for the survival of the Irish (Figure 41). The access we now enjoy to thousands of fruits and vegetables from the four corners of the earth is the direct result of the importance given to plants in the course of history and the considerable efforts that have been made to establish them as cornerstones of the human diet.

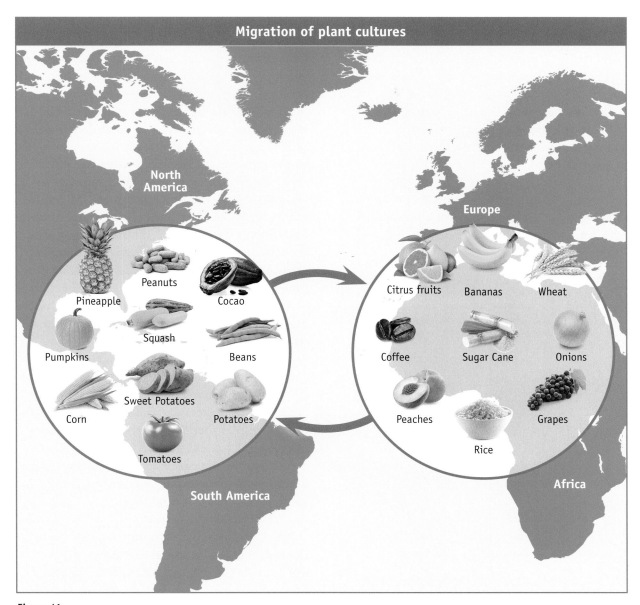

Figure 41

This love of fruits and vegetables is actually not that surprising: it must never be forgotten that even though we have become the most intelligent species to ever have lived on the planet, our metabolism — the way we absorb nutrients — is the legacy of our great ape ancestors, whose diet consisted almost exclusively of plants growing in their environment. Thus, even though we have gradually incorporated foods from animal sources into our diet in the course of evolution, our organism remains fundamentally dependent on plants to function at its best.

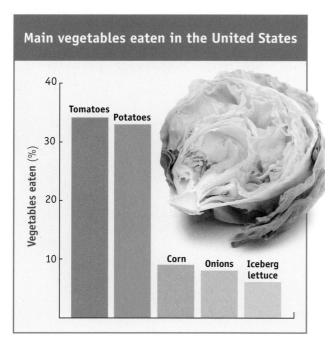

Main vegetables eaten in the United States

Tomatoes
Potatoes
Corn
Onions
Iceberg lettuce

Vegetables eaten (%)

40
30
20
10

Figure 42

Adapted from www.ers.usda.gov, 2013.

Plant Deficiency

Despite the importance of plants for health and the wide availability of fresh fruits and vegetables all year long, plant-based foods are still the most overlooked elements in the modern diet. All organizations dedicated to preventing chronic diseases, whether heart disease, diabetes or cancer, agree in saying that eating at least five servings (14 ounces, or 400 g) of fruits and vegetables a day is absolutely essential to reduce the incidence of these diseases and the mortality associated with them. Yet, despite this consensus, most people living in industrialized countries show little interest in these foods and consume nowhere near the recommended number of servings. In the United States, for example, 68% of adults eat fewer than two pieces of fruit per day and 74% eat fewer than three servings of vegetables daily. When this is compared to the total number of calories ingested, the situation is even worse, with fewer than 10% of people eating the recommended minimum of plants. Similar results have been observed in countries in economic transition, with 78% of people eating less than five servings of plant foods a day, a proportion that could even be as high as 99% in some countries, like Pakistan.

Not only are these amounts too low, but the plants eaten are not very varied and do not provide the maximum benefit from these foods. The eating habits of Americans are a revealing example in this regard, with most of their vegetable intake coming from the potatoes and tomatoes in fast-food meals (french fries and pizza), while corn, onions and some kinds of lettuce lag far behind (Figure 42). As paradoxical as it may seem, the overabundance of food typical of our era is accompanied by a severe deficiency in plant-based foods, the impact of which is accentuated by the low consumption of foods known to have the greatest positive benefits for health, for example cruciferous vegetables, whole grains and berries. In other words, we eat a lot, but not the way we should: too much sugar, fat and meat, and not enough fruits and vegetables. Correcting these extremes by putting plant-based products back in the forefront of our

diets is an essential prerequisite for any preventive approach aiming to lighten the load imposed by chronic diseases, including cancer.

Anticancer Cocktail

Plants are indispensable in preventing cancer because they are the only foods able to slow down the development of the microscopic tumors that form spontaneously during our lifetimes (see Chapter 1). Far from just being sources of vitamins and minerals, plants are also highly complex living organisms, whose metabolism produces an array of insecticide, bactericide and fungicide molecules that protect them from the many pathogens in the

Main food sources for various families of phytochemical compounds			
Family	Examples of molecules	Best sources	Contents (mg/100 g)
Polyphenols	Epigallocatechin gallate (EGCG)	Green tea	8,295
	Proanthocyanidins	Cacao	1,373
	Apigenin	Parsley	302
	Lignans	Flaxseed	300
	Ellagic acid	Raspberry	150
	Genistein	Soy (miso)	36
	Delphinidin	Blueberry	30
Sulfur compounds	PEITC	Watercress	400
	Sulforaphane	Broccoli	290
	Allicin	Garlic	4
Terpenes	Lycopene	Tomato (paste)	75
	Fucoxanthin	Wakame	32
	Zeaxanthin/lutein	Spinach	30

Figure 43

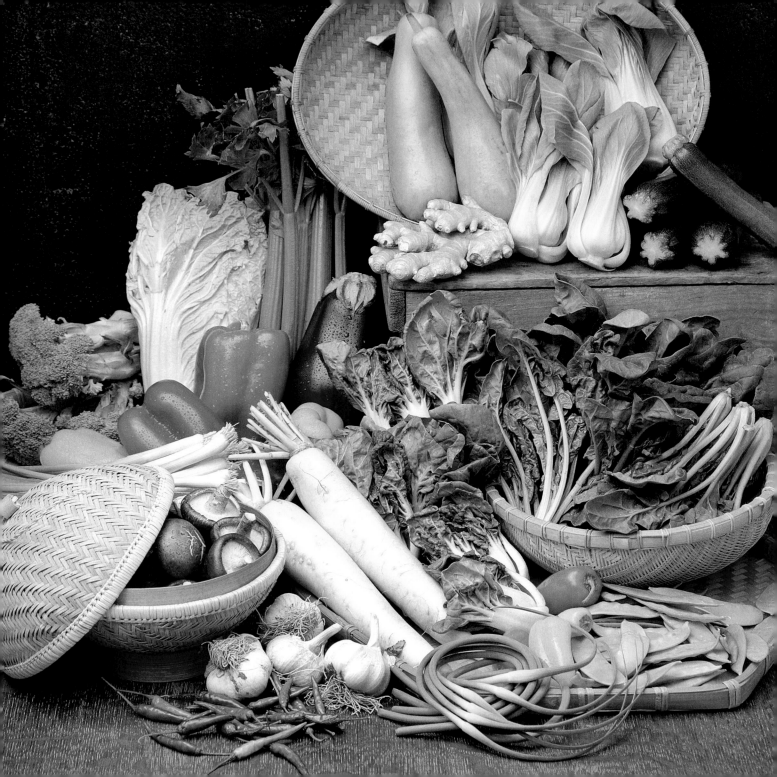

environment. The diversity of this arsenal is impressive, with over 10,000 distinct molecules identified to date, all belonging to one of the three main families of phytochemical compounds, either polyphenols, sulfur compounds (isothiocyanates and allyl sulfides), or terpenes (carotenoids and monoterpenes) (Figure 43).

As luck would have it, the beneficial action of these compounds is not limited to this plant defense effect: a great many studies have shown that a large number of these molecules have clearly defined pharmacological properties that interfere with several phenomena essential to the emergence and development of cancer cells in human beings (Figure 44).

For example, the sulfur compounds in garlic and in vegetables from the cabbage family prevent the activation of carcinogenic substances and speed up their elimination from the body, which reduces DNA damage and thus the occurrence of mutations that can facilitate

Main pharmacological targets for plant phytochemical compounds

Pharmacological target	Examples of molecules	Food source
Inhibition		
Tumor invasion and metastasis	Epigallocatechin gallate	Green tea
Growth factor receptors	Epigallocatechin gallate, delphinidin, ellagic acid	Green tea, blueberries, raspberries, nuts
Inflammatory response (NF$_\kappa$B, COX-2)	Curcumin, resveratrol	Turmeric, grapes
Chemotherapy resistance	Diallyl sulfide	Garlic
Angiogenesis	Epigallocatechin gallate	Green tea
Estrogenic actions	Genistein, lignans	Soy, flaxseed
Activation of carcinogens (Phase I enzymes)	Indole-3-carbinol	Cabbage
Activation		
Tumor cell apoptosis	Phenethyl isothiocyanate (PEITC)	Cress
Immune function	Lentinan, proanthocyanidins, lycopene	Shiitake, cacao, tomato
Carcinogen detoxification (Phase II enzymes)	Sulforaphane	Broccoli

Figure 44

cancer development. At the same time, certain polyphenols like epigallocatechin gallate in green tea or delphinidin in blueberries can neutralize cancer cells by halting their growth or preventing angiogenesis, the formation of a network of blood vessels required to supply oxygen and nutrients to these cells. These anticancer properties are made all the more effective by the fact that ingesting phytochemical compounds is also associated with a reduction in chronic inflammation, which deprives the precancerous lesions of a cellular environment favorable to the extra

mutations that would enable them to develop into a mature cancer. Consuming plant-based foods, whether fruits, vegetables, whole grains, spices and herbs, or beverages like green tea, is therefore not only an excellent way to supply the body with the vitamins and minerals essential for the optimal functioning of our cells, but also a kind of preventive chemotherapy through which the thousands of phytochemical compounds in these foods create an inhospitable environment for microscopic tumors and manage to keep them in a latent and harmless state.

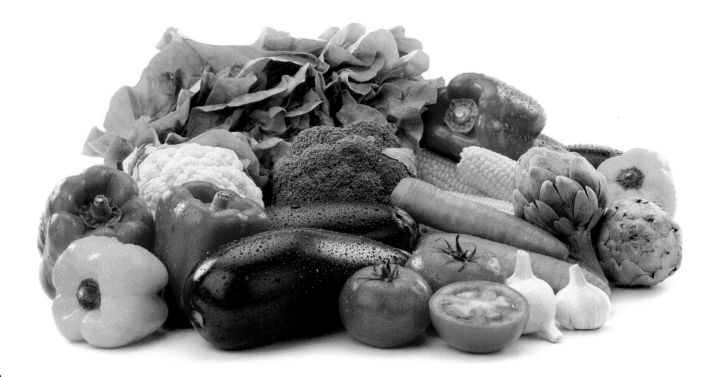

You Can Judge a Book by its Cover

The vital role of phytochemical compounds in preventing cancer means that only those plants containing the highest amounts can actually influence the chance of getting this disease. This is a very important concept, as plants are not a homogeneous class of foods: the phytochemical compound content of a head of lettuce or a potato cannot be compared with that of broccoli or green tea, any more than eating a banana means we absorb the same amount of anticancer molecules as are in a serving of blueberries. From a general health standpoint, there is no doubt that

it's important to increase overall fruit and vegetable intake to benefit from their vitamin, fiber and mineral content, and at the same time consume fewer high-calorie products. Furthermore, people who eat large amounts of plants, no matter which ones, reduce their heart disease risk by about 15%. To prevent cancer, on the other hand, it is actually the type of plants consumed daily that is key to significantly reducing the risk of developing the disease, as plant consumption as a whole is associated with only a slight decrease in risk, approximately 5 to 10%, whereas some fruits and vegetables can reduce risk for several types of cancer to a much greater degree (Figure 45).

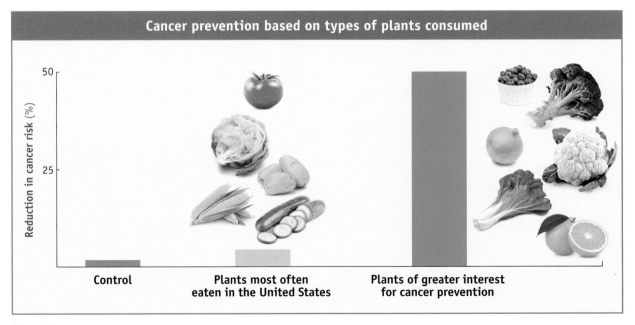

Figure 45

Eating the right kinds of fruits and vegetables is critical, but ensuring a varied intake of anticancer plants is also absolutely necessary to make the most of their chemopreventive potential. Cancer is a very complex disease, which uses various strategies to develop depending on the organ in which it is growing, and no food in and of itself has all the anticancer molecules needed to curtail the development of every cancer. Regular consumption of tomato-based products, for example, is known to significantly lower the risk of prostate cancer, but has no preventive effect against several other cancers (Figure 46). The same holds true for all food plants, even those with the highest amounts of anticancer molecules. Each class of food is only active against certain very specific cancers (Figure 47), and only by regularly eating a wide variety of plants with anticancer properties can these preventive actions be combined and the overall risk of cancer lowered.

The potential for cancer prevention (and prevention of chronic diseases in general) of an increased intake of plants is enormous. According to the World Health Organization (WHO), fruit and vegetable deficiency is directly responsible for roughly 3 million deaths every year worldwide, and up to 20% of esophageal and stomach cancers and 12% of lung cancers could be prevented by eating more of these plants. Such a reduction in the number of

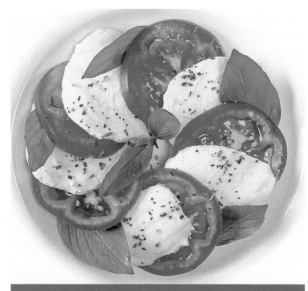

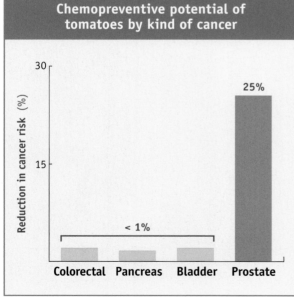

Chemopreventive potential of tomatoes by kind of cancer

Figure 46

cancer cases would obviously have major repercussions for life expectancy, since people who never eat fruits and vegetables have a 53% higher risk of dying prematurely and having a life span 3 years shorter than those who eat at least five servings a day. A recent study also indicates that people with the highest urinary concentrations of polyphenols, a marker for high plant-food intake, have a 30% lower risk of dying prematurely. These results are all the more remarkable given that these studies looked at plant consumption overall, without taking into account the specific intake of those known to have a powerful protective effect against heart disease and cancer (cruciferous vegetables, for example). It's therefore likely that people who eat a lot of these "super plants," containing large amounts of anti-inflammatory

and anticancer molecules, could see an even longer life expectancy.

It is also important to note that in all of these studies, the positive impact of plants was observed following the consumption of fruits and vegetables farmed with conventional agricultural methods — in other words, using pesticides to fight harmful insects or parasites. It's therefore not necessary to eat "organic" products to get the benefits of these foods, especially since no study has been able to show an increase in cancer risk related to tiny residual traces of these pesticides on plants.

That said, there are nonetheless excellent reasons for choosing plants grown organically. The absence of chemical fertilizers and

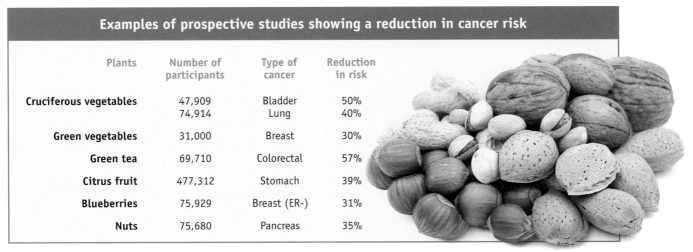

Examples of prospective studies showing a reduction in cancer risk

Plants	Number of participants	Type of cancer	Reduction in risk
Cruciferous vegetables	47,909	Bladder	50%
	74,914	Lung	40%
Green vegetables	31,000	Breast	30%
Green tea	69,710	Colorectal	57%
Citrus fruit	477,312	Stomach	39%
Blueberries	75,929	Breast (ER-)	31%
Nuts	75,680	Pancreas	35%

Figure 47

111

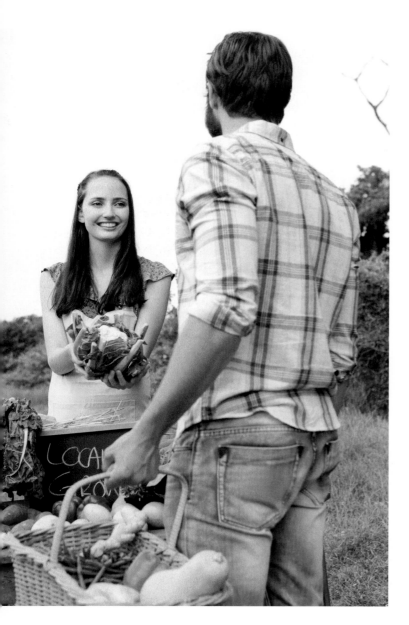

pesticides in organic farming reduces soil and water table contamination; it also reduces the exposure of some workers to very high amounts of these products that can increase their risk of getting a number of cancers (lymphoma, myeloma, prostate, kidney and lung cancer). We may also prefer organic products that seem to us to look better, taste better or that come from small local producers we want to support. Lastly, for people who are concerned about being exposed to particular environmental factors beyond their control, the idea of better controlling the contents of their plate by choosing products grown without chemical agents can be appealing. Buying organic fruits and vegetables must therefore be viewed as a personal choice, which may not have a major impact on our health, but which can have significant social and environmental repercussions.

Changing the modern diet so as to include more foods with higher levels of anticancer molecules, whether or not they are organic, is therefore a concrete way to lower the incidence of several types of cancer, including those hitting the populations of industrialized countries the hardest (colon, breast and prostate). Our current state of knowledge indicates that certain food families are especially promising in this respect.

Garlic and Its Cousins Keep Cancer at Bay!

Phytochemical compounds: allicin, diallyl sulfide, diallyl trisulfide

Main cancers: esophagus, stomach, colon

Garlic is perhaps the oldest example of a plant used as much for its nutritive properties as for its positive health effects. Considered by the Egyptians and Greeks to be a food that gave strength and endurance (the first Olympians consumed large amounts of garlic before their competitions, which makes it the first athletic performance-enhancing substance in history), garlic was also an indispensable ingredient in the traditional medicines of early civilizations, used since ancient times as a remedy for a wide variety of conditions, ranging from infections to circulation, respiratory or digestive problems.

A number of population studies indicate that people who regularly eat vegetables from the garlic family (garlic, onions, shallots, chives, leeks) have a lower risk of developing certain types of cancer, in particular cancers of the digestive system (stomach, esophagus, colon). A protective effect against cancers of the prostate, pancreas and breast has also been reported. Studies done on model systems indicate that these anticancer effects are due to sulfur compounds found in vegetables in this family, like diallyl sulfide and diallyl disulfide in garlic, or the sulfenic acid and thiosulfinates in onions. These molecules have the ability to block the formation of carcinogenic compounds (nitrosamines, for example) and limit the growth of several kinds of cancer cells.

Garlic and its close relatives are clearly indispensable plants for preventing cancer, and they should be eaten as regularly as possible. The WHO recommends that adults eat $1/12$ to $1/6$ ounce (2–5 g) of fresh garlic daily, or approximately one clove.

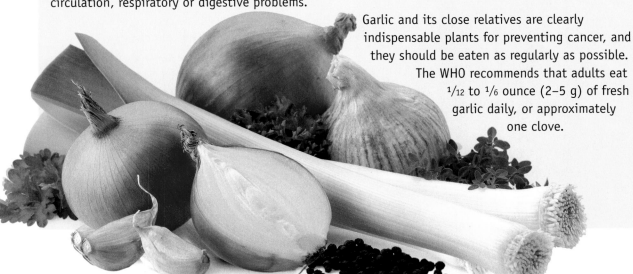

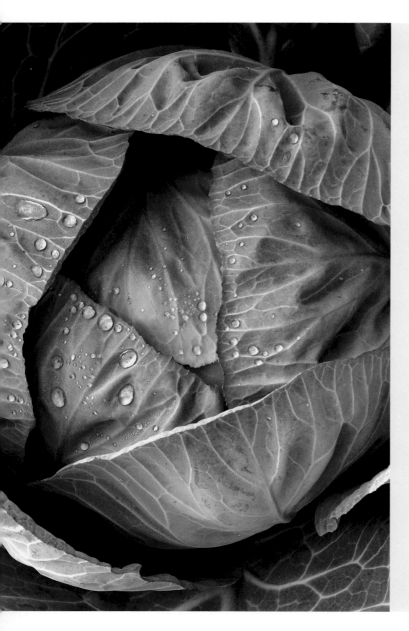

The Cruciferous Vegetables, Crossing Out Cancer

Phytochemical compounds: sulforaphane, PEITC, I3C

Main cancers: lung, bladder, prostate

The crucifers are a family of plants that produce flowers with four petals in the shape of a Greek cross. Different varieties of cabbage, broccoli, cauliflower, radish and turnip are the crucifers eaten most often, but cress, arugula and rapini are also part of this family and provide an opportunity to enjoy the benefits of cruciferous vegetables while adding variety to the meals we prepare.

The crucifers are one of the most studied plant families, having been the subject of more than 20,000 scientific articles in recent decades. The importance of these vegetables in preventing cancer stems from the fact that they are the only food plants to contain large amounts of glucosinolates, a class of inert compounds that are changed into powerful anticancer molecules (isothiocyanates and indoles) when plant cells are broken down by chewing.

The regular consumption of cruciferous vegetables is associated with a significant reduction in risk for several types of cancer. This protective effect is especially well documented in the case of lung cancer (even in smokers), bladder cancer and prostate cancer, but recent studies suggest that these vegetables might also lower the risk of colon, stomach and breast cancer. In the latter case, eating one serving of a cruciferous vegetable daily resulted in a 50% drop in cancer risk in Chinese women, whereas a weekly serving of these vegetables reduced this risk by 17% in a European population (Italy and Switzerland).

Practical suggestions

Increasing the consumption of cruciferous vegetables is all the more important because it's so low in most western countries, barely $9/10$ to 1 ounce (25–30 g) a day, compared with more than $3\frac{1}{2}$ ounces (100 g) in China. Some isothiocyanates, especially sulforaphane in broccoli and 2-phenethyl isothiocyanate (PEITC) in watercress, have particularly powerful anticancer properties, and including these two vegetables in the diet can't help but maximize the chemopreventive effect of cruciferous vegetables.

The best way to get the full benefits of the anticancer properties of cruciferous vegetables is to steam or sauté them, to optimize their isothiocyanate content. Exceptionally for this vegetable family, frozen products should be avoided as much as possible, since the blanching at high temperature required to preserve vegetables renders the myrosinase inactive. That said, recent research indicates that adding radish extract to these vegetables will compensate for the loss of this enzyme, and these frozen products might therefore deserve a second look in the near future.

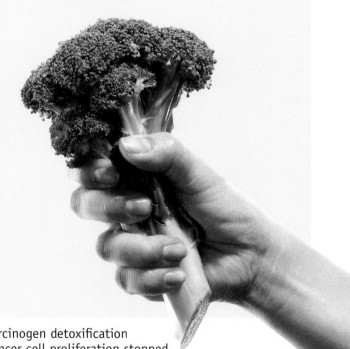

Myrosinase

Glucosinolates ⟶ Isothiocyanates ⟨ Carcinogen detoxification
Cancer cell proliferation stopped
Death of cancer cells

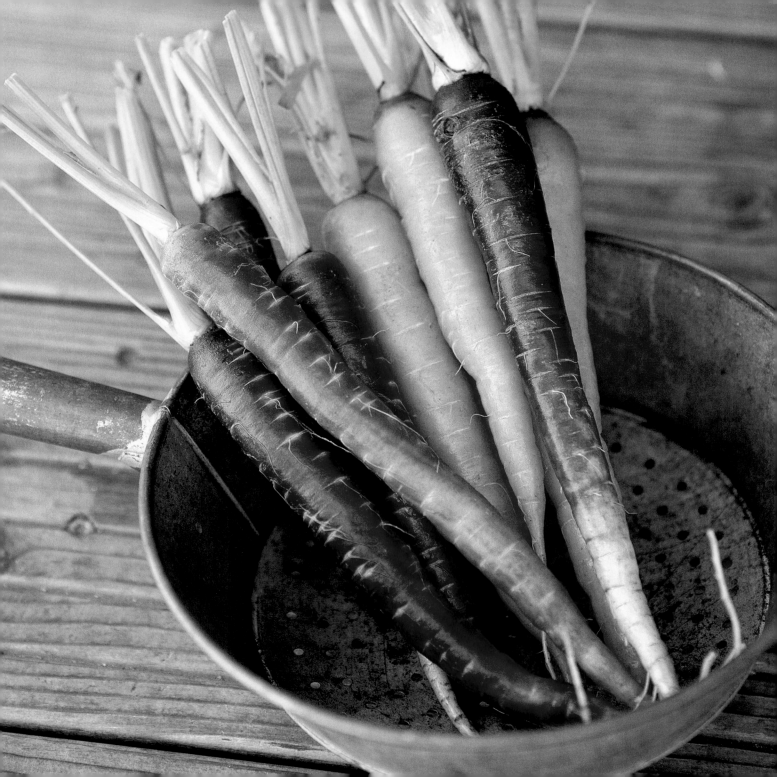

Carotenoids, Adding Color to Cancer Prevention!

Phytochemical compounds: lycopene, beta-carotene, lutein, fucoxanthin

Main cancers: prostate, lung, breast

Carotenoids are natural pigments responsible for the colors ranging from orangey-yellow to purplish-red in a wide variety of fruits and vegetables. Although there are more than 600 different carotenoids, beta-carotene (carrots), lutein (spinach) and lycopene (tomatoes) alone make up nearly 80% of the total.

Lycopene is the carotenoid whose anticancer activity has been best established. Regular consumption of tomato-based products is associated with a reduction in prostate cancer risk of roughly 25%, a protection that can even reach 53% for advanced forms of this disease. The anticancer effect of lycopene is mainly observed in men 65 and over who do not have any family history of prostate cancer. The other dietary carotenoids are not to be discounted, since a high intake of alpha- and beta-carotene, as well as lutein, is associated with a significant drop in the risk for hormone-independent (ER-) breast cancer, as well as lung cancer. In the latter instance, it's interesting to note that the inhabitants of the Fiji Islands, who eat large amounts of green vegetables high in lutein, have a lower incidence of lung cancer than other Pacific populations whose diet does not include many carotenoid-rich plants. This anticancer activity is not limited to "land" fruits and vegetables; laboratory studies indicate that the fucoxanthin in algae is a powerful anticancer agent, which might contribute to the exceptional longevity of the inhabitants of Okinawa, who eat these foods daily.

Practical suggestions

Eating whole fruits and vegetables is essential to getting the most benefit from carotenoids, as several studies have shown that supplements containing large amounts of beta-carotene do not have protective effects against cancer and may even increase the incidence of lung cancer in people at risk (smokers or workers exposed to asbestos).

On the other hand, unlike a number of other plant components that can be destroyed by heat, the bioavailability of carotenoids (found in the chloroplasts of plants, where they are closely linked to other molecules) increases when these structures are broken down during cooking. These molecules are also not very water-soluble, and they can often be more easily absorbed in the presence of fatty substances.

Small Fruits, Big Benefits

Phytochemical compounds: anthocyanins (delphinidin), ellagic acid

Main cancer: breast

Strawberries, blueberries and raspberries are exceptional sources of anticancer phytochemical compounds capable of interfering in several processes involved in the growth and potential invasiveness of cancer cells. Polyphenols like delphinidin (blueberries) and ellagic acid (raspberries and strawberries) hinder the formation of a new blood vessel network around tumors (angiogenesis), thus depriving them of oxygen and nutritive molecules. Recent studies indicate that the phytochemical compounds in blueberries interfere with cell growth in triple-negative breast cancer. To inhibit the development of this cancer, a 130-pound (60 kg) woman requires approximately 3½ ounces (100 g) of blueberries a day, an amount easily obtained through diet. In addition, a clinical study recently showed that eating just one serving of blueberries a week led to a 31% reduction in hormone-independent breast cancer risk in menopausal women. Blueberries may also have an indirect positive effect on cancer risk by specifically keeping preadipocytes from turning into mature adipocytes, reducing fat accumulation and preventing obesity from developing. As well, an analysis of the dietary habits of more than 200,000 Americans has shown that people who eat two servings weekly of anthocyanin-rich foods, especially blueberries, have a 25% lower risk of developing type 2 diabetes and are therefore less exposed to the increased cancer risk that accompanies chronic hyperglycemia.

The phytochemical compounds in berries also reach the colon, where they are metabolized by bacterial flora and might act locally to prevent colorectal cancer.

Practical suggestions

Since the berry season is relatively short, berries are commonly preserved for later use. Freezing the whole fruit is considered the best way to preserve both its shape and its phytochemical compound content. Making jams also works well; an analysis of the polyphenols in strawberries preserved in this way showed no significant loss even after 5 months of storage at 77°F (25°C). Prolonged cooking of berries and their subsequent storage, in the form of pies, for example, may not be the best technique, as it results in a significant reduction in their anthocyanin content.

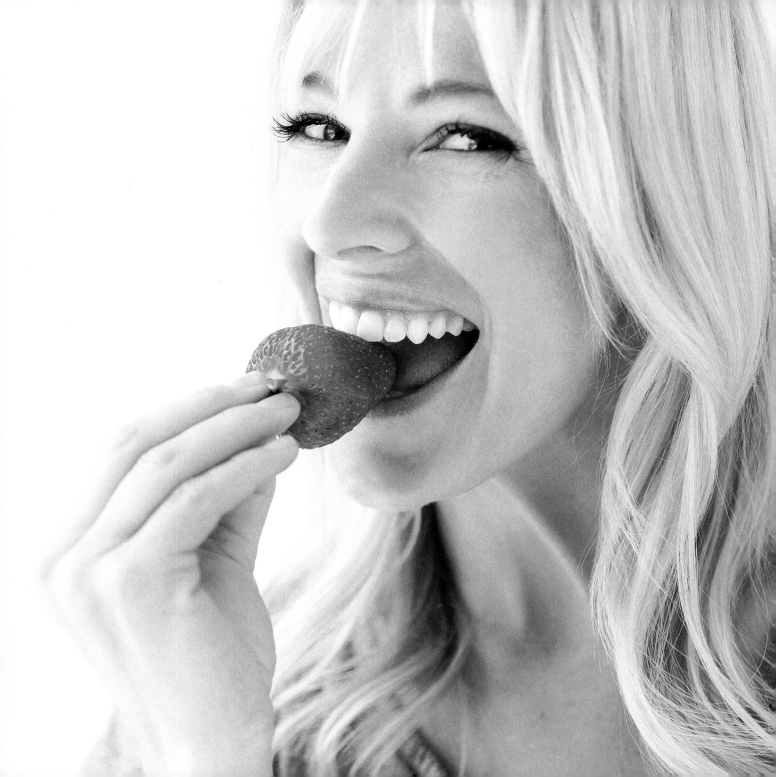

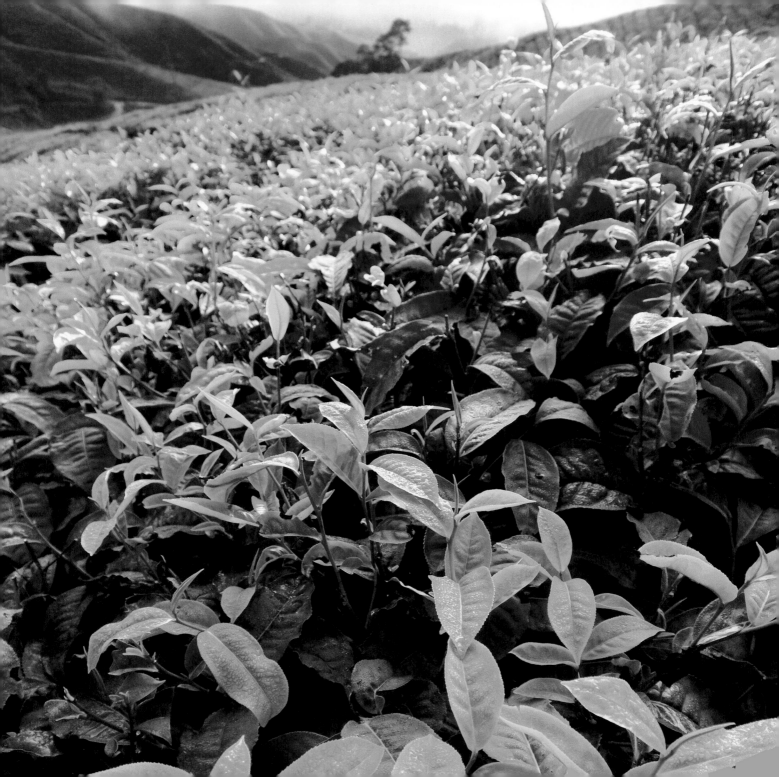

Green Tea

Phytochemical compound: epigallocatechin gallate

Main cancers: colon, stomach

Of all the plants that are part of the human diet, the leaves of *Camellia sinensis* contain the highest proportion of anticancer molecules. A single cup of green tea can have up to 200 mg of polyphenols (flavonols, phenolic acids, catechins), notably epigallocatechin gallate (ECGC), the main molecule responsible for this tea's beneficial effects.

Over 11,000 scientific studies have shown that ECGC is a polyvalent molecule that can interfere in a wide range of processes used by cancer cells to grow and invade organs. The importance of these many biological activities is clearly illustrated by the marked decrease in risk for several cancers associated with the regular consumption of green tea, especially those that attack the organs in the digestive system (stomach, esophagus and colon), a decrease that can be as high as 60%. Decreases of 20% in lung cancer risk (in nonsmokers), 50% for prostate cancer and 40% for breast cancer have also been observed, confirming the inhibiting effect of tea on the development of these cancers in experimental models.

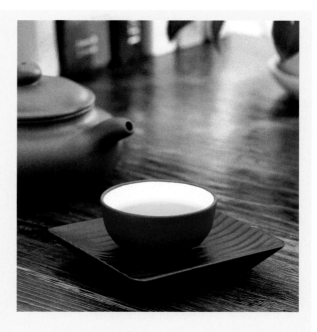

Practical suggestions

Japanese green teas, higher in catechins, are the best source of ECGC, especially if the leaves are infused for 8 to 10 minutes to extract the most polyphenols. These molecules are associated with a mellow bitterness, a taste not very familiar to westerners, but which it is important to learn to appreciate to get the most benefit from the anticancer properties of the plant's phytochemical compounds. It is however best to avoid drinking the tea too hot, as overly high temperatures seem to cancel out the decrease in stomach cancer risk observed in people who regularly drink this beverage.

A Handful of Nuts a Day Keeps the Doctor Away

Phytochemical compounds: linolenic acid, phenolic compounds

Main cancers: breast, colon, prostate, pancreas

Oleaginous fruits and seeds are outstanding foods that have for too long been ignored because of the phobia about everything containing fat. Yet this may be one of the classes of foods with the most beneficial effects on health. Several observations indicate that simply eating three servings of nuts a week can reduce the risk of premature death by about 30% by significantly lowering the risk of heart disease, type 2 diabetes, respiratory illnesses and cancer. In the latter case, a protective effect against colon and prostate cancers has been suggested and could be due to nuts' high levels of anti-inflammatory omega-3s, fiber and phenolic compounds. Recently, regularly eating nuts (twice a week) has been associated with a sizable drop in pancreatic cancer risk, perhaps because it prevents type 2 diabetes, a major cancer risk factor.

Practical suggestions

Many people refrain from eating nuts on the pretext that they contain a lot of calories. Yet studies indicate that eating nuts is actually associated with a lower obesity risk. From a botanical standpoint, walnuts, hazelnuts, chestnuts and pecans are the only true representatives of this family, but in practice, the term "nut" also includes almonds, cashews, Brazil nuts, macadamia nuts and pine nuts, pistachios and peanuts. All of these fruits make outstanding snacks with positive health effects we are often unaware of, although these foods have been part of our daily lives forever. For example, a study indicates that girls who regularly eat peanut butter have a 40% lower risk of developing benign proliferative breast disease, lesions that significantly increase cancer risk.

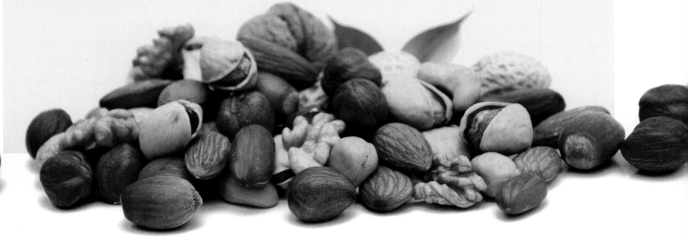

Soy, an Anticancer Legume

Phytochemical compound: genistein

Main cancer: breast

Soy beans are a major source of isoflavones, a class of phytoestrogens that interfere with the growth of hormone-dependent cancers, especially those of the breast and prostate. With regard to breast cancer, currently available data indicate that consuming soy during childhood and adolescence reduces cancer risk the most, which would explain, at least in part, the dramatic gap between the incidence of this cancer in Asia and in the West. A lower endometrial cancer risk, as well as lower lung cancer risk, has also been observed, showing the degree to which incorporating soy into the diet, especially during childhood, can have extraordinary effects on cancer risk.

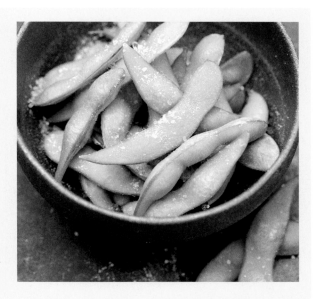

In recent years, the consumption of soy-based products, especially supplements, by women with breast cancer has raised a number of questions, but a large number of recent studies show unequivocally that soy is not dangerous and might even be linked to a significant decrease in the risk of recurrence (see p. 235).

Practical suggestions

Soy isoflavones occur in large amounts in fresh beans (edamame), tofu and miso, and these foods are all simple, quick and economical ways to benefit from the anticancer properties of these molecules. Industrial products made with soy protein concentrates, however, are lacking in isoflavones and play no role in preventing cancer.

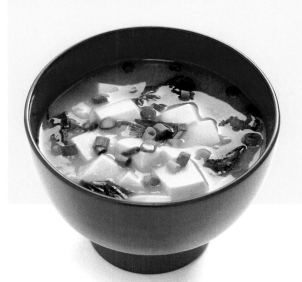

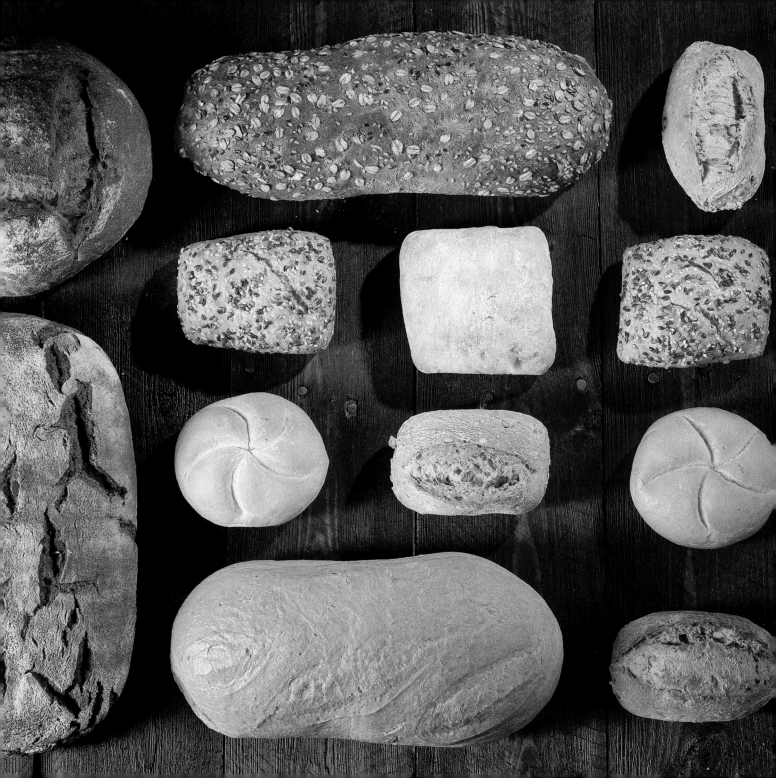

Seeds and Grains

Phytochemical compounds: linolenic acid, lignans (secoisolariciresinol, matairesinol)

Main cancers: breast, colon

Just like nuts, flaxseeds are an outstanding source of anti-inflammatory short-chain omega-3s, and consuming them regularly is likely to help reduce chronic inflammation and create an environment resistant to cancer cell development. Patients with prostate cancer have seen the growth of their cancer slow down significantly after eating 1 ounce (30 g) of ground flaxseeds daily.

Flaxseeds, like whole grains, also contain phenomenal amounts of lignans, a class of phytoestrogens distinct from soy isoflavones. Studies have led us to conclude that eating flaxseeds or bread containing them is associated with an approximately 20% decrease in breast cancer risk, in line with the protective effect of lignans from other plant sources. This decreased risk may be correlated with reduced inflammation, as the presence of large amounts of urinary lignans is accompanied by a decrease in several inflammatory markers.

Practical suggestions

The decrease in breast cancer risk observed after eating flaxseeds calls for only about 5 mg of lignans, an amount easily obtained in the diet (13 mg of lignans per teaspoon of flaxseeds). Adding these seeds to yogurt and breakfast cereals, or when baking cakes, muffins or bread, is therefore an easy and inexpensive way to get the benefits of flax. Products made from whole grains — bread, cereals, pasta — are also a good idea, for in addition to having significant amounts of lignans, these foods are major sources of fiber and can thus play an undeniable role in colorectal cancer prevention.

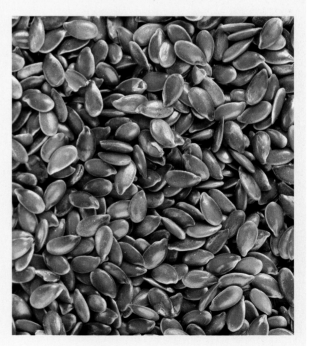

Olive Oil, the Soul of the Mediterranean Diet

Phytochemical compounds: oleic acid, oleocanthal, hydroxytyrosol, taxifolin

Main cancer: colon

The diet of people living around the Mediterranean Sea has a number of positive effects on health, especially for the prevention of heart disease and several types of cancer. This should actually come as no surprise, since theirs is an exemplary diet, high in fruits and vegetables, as well as in monounsaturated and polyunsaturated omega-3 fatty acids; the complex sugars in fiber and grains are the main sources of carbohydrates in this diet and the protein comes mainly from fish and legumes, rather than red meat.

Population studies have shown that people who follow a Mediterranean-style diet have a roughly 15% lower risk of getting cancer. Olive oil is the cornerstone of this type of diet, and recent results suggest that it might contribute to cancer prevention. This oil contains oleocanthal, an anti-inflammatory molecule not unlike ibuprofen that might therefore have similar effects in preventing colon cancer. In addition, at least two phenolic compounds found in large amounts in olive oil, hydroxytyrosol and taxifolin, effectively inhibit the formation of new blood vessels and might as a result slow down the development of a large array of cancers.

Practical suggestions

Choosing virgin or extra-virgin oils is essential, both for their superior taste and for their health benefits. These oils contain the polyphenols from the original olives; this is easy to recognize, as one of these polyphenols, oleocanthal, causes a tickling or tingling sensation in the throat, a pungency resulting from its specific interaction with certain receptors in the larynx. The more it tingles, the more powerful the olive oil's anti-inflammatory action!

Citrus fruits

Phytochemical compounds: monoterpenes, flavanones

Main cancer: stomach

Especially known for their high vitamin C content, citrus fruits also contain several phytochemical compounds — polyphenols and monoterpenes that can help prevent cancer. Laboratory studies suggest that these molecules act against several kinds of cancer cells, and epidemiological data indicate that the regular consumption of citrus fruits is associated with a decreased risk of stomach and esophageal cancer.

Citrus fruits also influence cancer risk indirectly, by regulating the enzyme systems involved in eliminating foreign substances from the body. Grapefruit, for example, is well known for blocking the cytochrome P450 systems; this cytochrome inhibition can prevent anticancer compounds from being eliminated too quickly, thus enhancing their action against precancerous lesions.

Practical suggestions

Since citrus fruits are very often consumed as juices, it must be remembered that these drinks are very sugary, and the lack of fiber means that the glucose and fructose they contain is absorbed very quickly. Rediscovering the pleasure of eating an orange or grapefruit is therefore a good way to get the benefits of these exceptional fruits while avoiding blood sugar fluctuations that are too sudden and can contribute to excess weight gain.

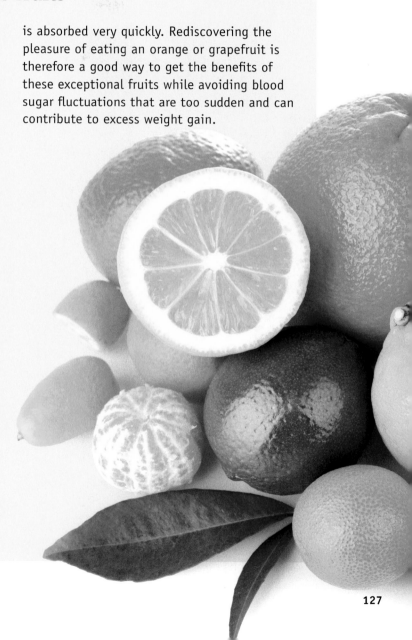

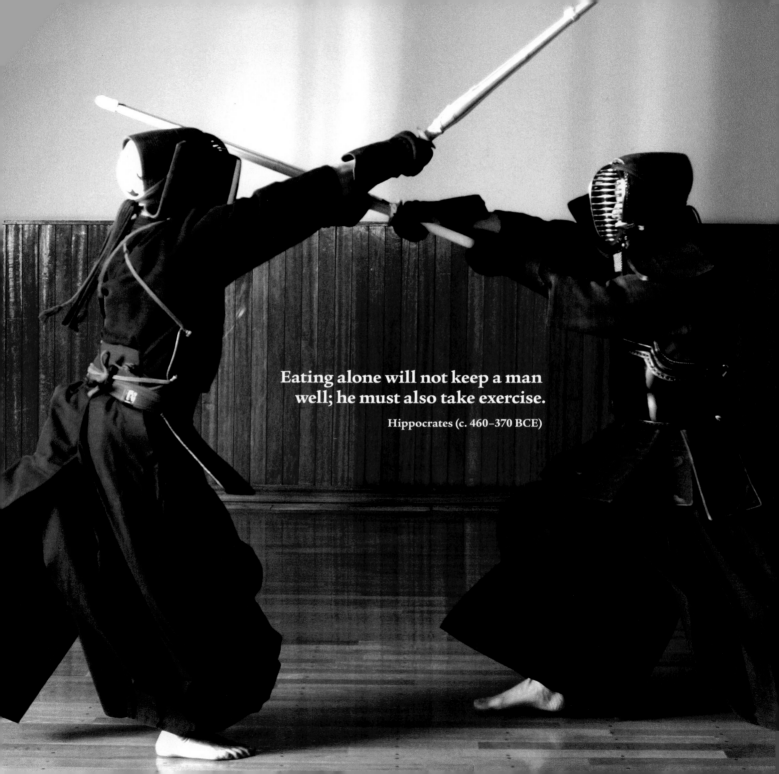

Eating alone will not keep a man
well; he must also take exercise.

Hippocrates (c. 460–370 BCE)

Chapter 6

Physical Exercise: Movement and Cancer Prevention

For fun, the Native American Rarámuri people of Mexico's Sierra Madre have for centuries participated in rarajipari competitions: the participants can run for more than 20 hours without once stopping, covering hundreds of miles while kicking and relentlessly pursuing a small wooden ball. Considered to be "the game of life" by the Rarámuri because of its difficulty and the uncertainty about when it will end, this ritual race is really an illustration of our inborn capacity for physical effort, as well as of the remarkable endurance of the human body. For although *Homo sapiens* holds a special place in the animal world because of his unequaled intellectual abilities, he remains fundamentally a *Homo activus,* endowed with a physiology that is perfectly adapted to intense physical activity. It must not be forgotten that the reason we have become so intelligent is simply because our body adapted to walking and running long distances, up to 12½ miles (20 km) a day on average, to obtain high-quality food with enough calories to meet the energy needs required for optimal functioning and the evolution of our large brain. We are not born just to think and innovate, but also, and perhaps especially, to move.

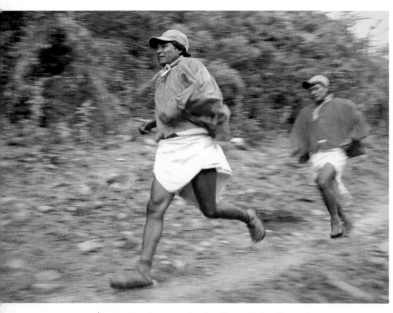

^ Rarámuri runners in the Sierra Madre (Mexico).

Muscles at Rest

The human body's biological predisposition to move has, however, largely fallen into disuse in the modern era. With the exception of high-performance athletes or people whose work is physically demanding (laborers, fire fighters, soldiers), most inhabitants of industrialized countries have to make very little physical effort in the course of their work or their daily tasks. In Canada, for example, barely 15% of the population gets at least 150 minutes of moderate physical activity per week, a proportion that drops even lower in people aged 60 and over. On average, adults spend nearly 10 of their waking hours every day on sedentary activities involving no physical effort.

This situation reflects major social changes rooted in industrialization and, more recently, the technological revolution: motorized means of transport make it possible to cover long distances without effort, the computer occupies a central place in an ever-increasing number of professions, and a series of new electronic devices continues to reduce the energy expenditure of our smallest actions and activities. This even applies to our leisure activities: the remote allows us to control the television without getting up, we can order and receive an item without having to leave the house, or rent a highly anticipated movie with a simple click of the remote or mouse. Worldwide, it's estimated that people burn on average 500 fewer calories a day than barely a century ago, a decrease that is all the more paradoxical given that dietary calorie intake has considerably increased during this period.

These advances are usually considered to be positive, with the backbreaking labor of days gone by replaced by activities that are much less physically exhausting, and modern technology lets us save time, precious time that we can devote to enhancing our productivity at work or our overall quality of life. This is, however, a trap, for although the material advantages technology offers are undeniable, the inactivity or immobility that results from these advances runs counter to our body's basic needs: the 640 or so muscles and 206 bones, which alone account for half of our body mass, have not been selected during evolution for us to remain seated in a car or in front of a computer or television for most of the day! After having been active

for 200,000 years, we have become sedentary in barely 50 and it's now obvious that this sudden change in our lifestyle habits is having negative repercussions on our bodies. Whether we like it or not, we still have the physiology we inherited from cave dwellers, but we live in a metabolically passive environment we are not suited to, and experience the side effects on health that this maladaptation can cause.

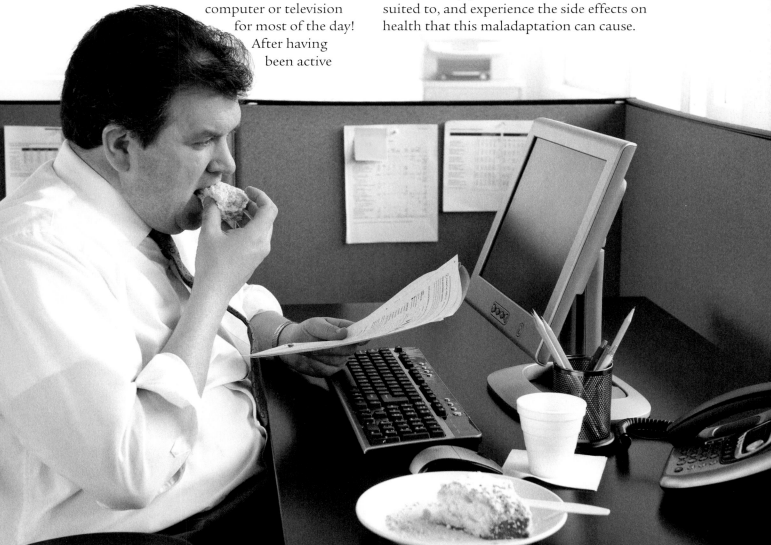

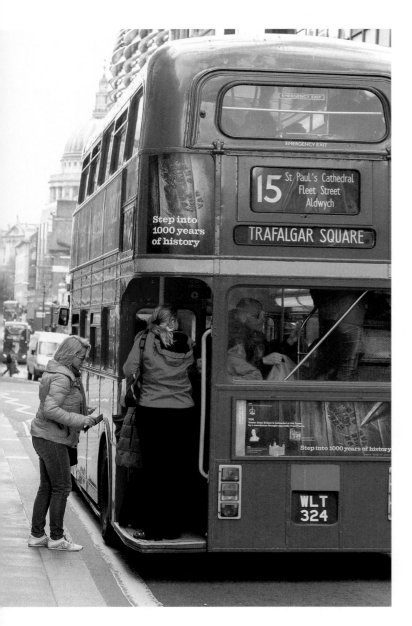

Putting Your Heart Into It

One of the first pieces of evidence pointing to the dangers inherent in a sedentary way of life came from the work of Britain's Jeremy Morris (1910–2009) on the incidence of heart disease in bus conductors and drivers on London's double-decker buses in 1953. He observed that conductors, who went up and down as many as 750 steps every day, had a 50% lower risk of heart disease than their driver colleagues, who spent more than 90% of their shifts sitting down. The same was true of British postal service employees: the carriers who delivered the mail on foot or by bicycle had far fewer heart problems than employees who worked at wickets.

We now know that the positive effect of exercise on the heart is due to a series of physiological and metabolic adaptations in the pulmonary, muscular and cardiovascular systems that, together, increase oxygen consumption and energy production. Lower blood pressure, an improved blood lipid profile, less inflammation and greater vessel elasticity resulting from exercise truly make it an all-in-one drug that targets several processes indispensable to maintaining cardiovascular health. What's more, recent studies indicate that physical activity is as effective as many drugs in reducing the mortality rate among people with coronary heart disease and those recovering from stroke.

In contrast to what many people might think, the benefits of physical activity are not limited to heart function or improved muscle tone. In recent years, a wide array of very beneficial effects have been closely linked to regular physical activity, which makes it the aspect of lifestyle that can have the greatest positive effect on health (Figure 48). And let's not forget that exercise causes the release of hormones in the brain like endorphins and endocannabinoids that "reward" active people by stimulating the neuronal circuits involved in the pleasure sensation, somewhat like a euphoria-inducing drug.

Cancer Likes Peace and Quiet

Of all the positive impacts of regular physical activity, cancer prevention remains the least well known. Yet a large number of studies have clearly shown that people who are the most physically active see their risk of getting several cancers drop considerably, compared with those who have a sedentary way of life. This protective effect is especially well documented for colon and breast cancer, with average risk reductions of 25% observed in dozens of studies, but some data suggest that endometrial, ovarian, lung and prostate cancer are also less common in active people (Figure 49). The reduction in cancer development associated with regular physical activity is

due to a combination of several hormonal, metabolic and immune-system factors.

Being physically active does not just mean getting our muscles moving; above all, activity causes a series of biochemical and physiological changes that create an environment that is inhospitable to precancerous cells and interferes with their development into advanced cancer. One of the most important effects of physical activity is to reduce chronic inflammation inside the body, thus depriving still immature cancer cells of a tool indispensable for their growth.

Main benefits of regular physical activity

- Lower diabetes risk
- Increased bone mass and prevention of osteoporosis
- Increased brain metabolism and prevention of neurodegenerative diseases
- Lower risk of getting certain cancers
- Less stress, sounder sleep and maintenance of immune function
- Greater self-confidence and resilience
- Enhanced sexual function
- Lower risk of depression

Figure 48

The muscles of active people also absorb blood sugar in response to insulin much more effectively, enabling the pancreas to secrete lower amounts of this hormone and reduce its harmful effects on the growth of cancer cells. As well, the lower steroid hormone level observed in physically active people seems to contribute to the prevention of cancers whose development is stimulated by these hormones, notably estrogen-dependent breast cancer. Nor should we ignore the positive effect of regular physical activity on the control of body weight; active people are usually slimmer than those who are sedentary. And too much fat significantly increases the risk of cancer because of the overproduction of inflammatory molecules, insulin and sex hormones (see Chapter 3).

All of these factors make physical activity an indispensable ingredient for preventing cancer, but its potential remains largely untapped in industrialized societies, where most people are physically inactive.

TV Can Be Deadly

In addition to depriving the body of the positive effects of physical activity, a sedentary lifestyle can cause health problems of its own, independent of those caused by lack of exercise. Being sedentary is associated with major metabolic disturbances, especially with regard to fat and blood sugar absorption, and is a significant risk factor for obesity and

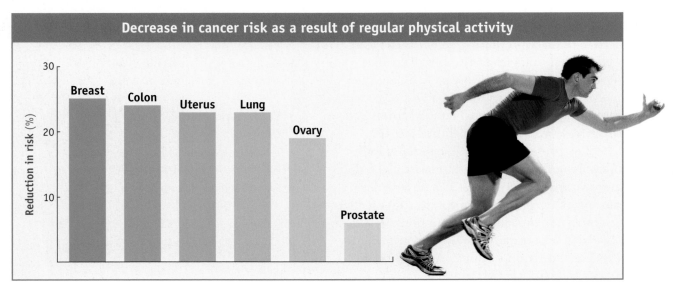

Decrease in cancer risk as a result of regular physical activity

Reduction in risk (%)

Breast Colon Uterus Lung Ovary Prostate

Figure 49

Adapted from Brown et al., 2012.

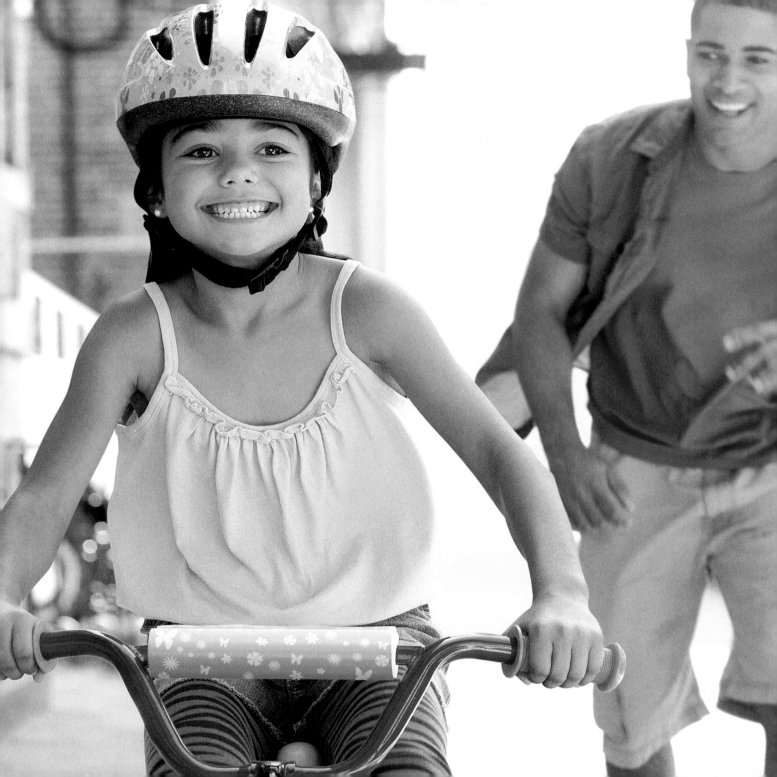

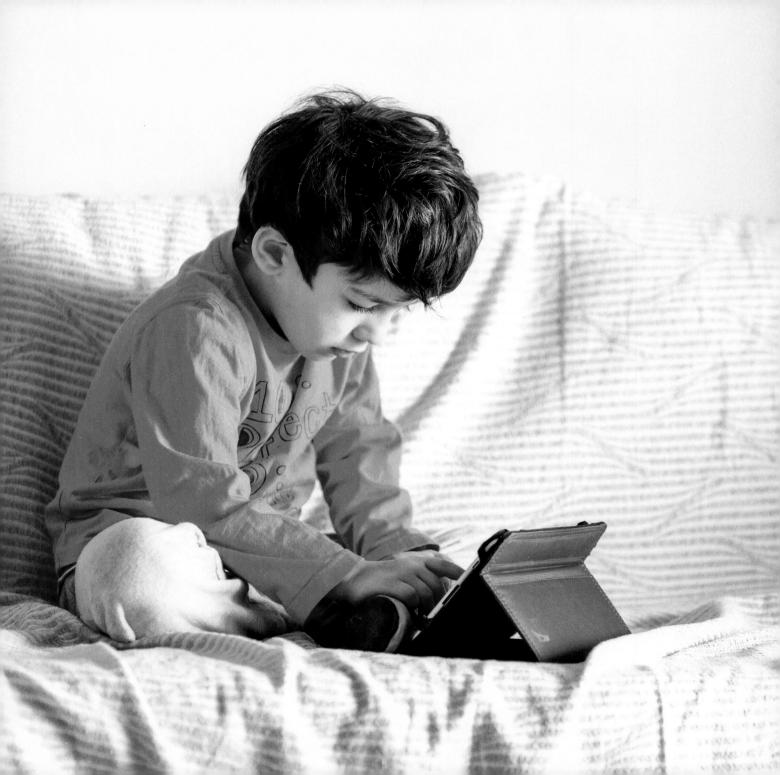

various chronic diseases. Several studies have shown that the time devoted to sedentary activities correlates with increased premature mortality risk. For example, people who spend more than 7 hours in front of the TV daily have an 85% higher risk of dying prematurely of heart disease and a 22% higher risk of dying from cancer than those who watch less than 1 hour a day. A complete analysis of all the studies done to date indicates that the risk for all chronic diseases is increased by physical inactivity, with this effect being especially pronounced for breast and colon cancer (Figure 50). A meta-analysis of nearly 69,000 people with cancer indicates that the number of hours spent in a sitting position is also associated with an increased risk of endometrial cancer (66%) and lung cancer (21%). It's estimated that up to 10% of these cancers could be prevented by eliminating a sedentary way of life, a protective effect that could have extraordinary repercussions, given the high incidence of these cancers in the West. Worldwide, lack of physical activity increases the risk of premature mortality by 28%; every year, it's directly responsible for over 5 million deaths around the world, as many as smoking.

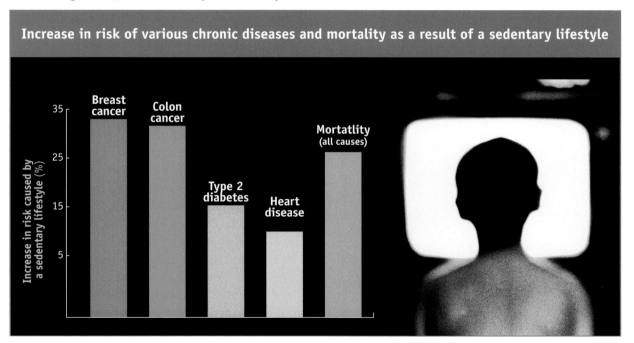

Increase in risk of various chronic diseases and mortality as a result of a sedentary lifestyle

Breast cancer
Colon cancer
Type 2 diabetes
Heart disease
Mortatlity (all causes)

Increase in risk caused by a sedentary lifestyle (%)

35
25
15
5

Figure 50

Adapted from Lee et al., 2012.

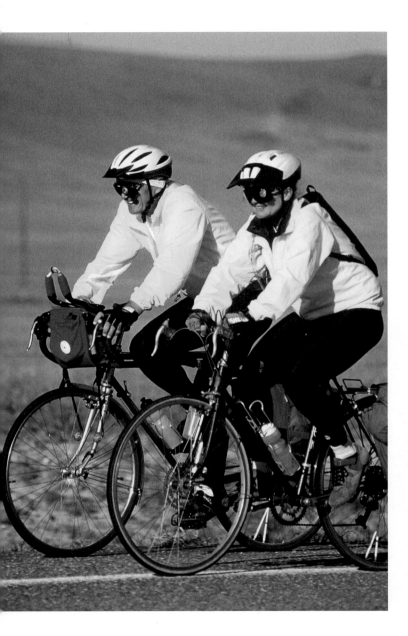

Active, but Sedentary

In Canada, as in most industrialized countries, people are advised to get at least 150 minutes of moderate- to vigorous-intensity physical activity per week to reap the health benefits. Although this is a minimum, only 15% of the population follow these recommendations, and barely 5% do so regularly, by being active at least 30 minutes a day, 5 days a week. Although following these recommendations is essential for preventing cancer and other chronic diseases, it's important to understand that a decrease in sedentary activities is also necessary. This may seem paradoxical, but in the world we live in it's entirely possible to reach a certain level of physical activity, theoretically adequate to reduce the risk of chronic disease, while remaining too sedentary. For example, a person can take a fast half-hour walk every morning (and thus follow the recommendations of 150 minutes of physical activity per week), but if he or she spends all day sitting in an office and then the evening in front of the TV before going to bed, he or she may be devoting more than 16 waking hours to passive activities. In other words, someone considered to be active, according to current criteria, may in fact only be active for 3% of their available time! In this kind of situation, the positive effects associated with 30 minutes of physical activity are in large part canceled out by the negative impact of a sedentary lifestyle on the metabolism. Furthermore, the increased mortality risk observed in people who spend many hours every week watching television is seen even in those who are physically active more than 7 hours a week. It's therefore critical to be physically active at least 30 minutes a day to prevent cancer, but to be of maximum value, this energy expenditure must go hand in hand with a broader change in lifestyle, in which time spent on sedentary activities is also reduced to a minimum.

Homo activus

Given the way work and leisure are organized nowadays, adopting a sufficiently active way of life to prevent cancer is a challenge that cannot be taken lightly. We have to start by being honest, since most of us have a tendency to overestimate our level of physical activity. For example, a recent poll indicates that 73% of Americans see themselves as being physically active, whereas only 15% of them actually are.

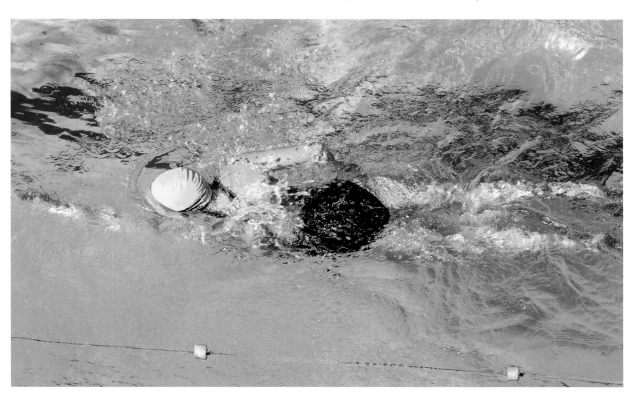

Physical Activity or Exercise?

Physical activity is usually defined as any movement that burns calories, whether during work or in carrying out daily tasks. Exercise, on the other hand, is considered to be a category of physical activity, usually done in periods of leisure, and whose goal is to improve the physical shape and health of the person who does it. In other words, washing the dishes is a physical activity, whereas jogging or playing tennis are forms of exercise.

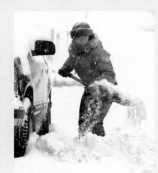

The intensity of these various kinds of physical activity is expressed in metabolic equivalents (METs); a MET is the metabolic cost (oxygen consumption) of the physical activity. One MET equals a resting metabolism (about $\frac{1}{9}$ fluid ounce or 3.5 ml of O_2/kg/minute, or 1 kcal/kg of body weight/hour). A person doing light physical activity "burns" up to three times more energy per minute than an inactive person, whereas moderate- and high-intensity activities are demanding enough to cause a calorie expenditure three to six times greater than in a seated person, respectively.

Various kinds of physical activity

Light physical activity (< 3.0 METs)
(METs: metabolic equivalents)

- Walking slowly
- Working seated at the computer
- Working standing up, performing activities like cooking or washing dishes
- Fishing sitting down
- Playing most musical instruments

Moderate physical activity (3.0–6.0 METs)

- Walking quickly
- Tidying or cleaning (washing windows, vacuuming or mopping)
- Mowing the lawn with an electric mower
- Cycling, medium effort
- Playing badminton
- Playing tennis (doubles)

Vigorous physical activity (> 6.0 METs)

- Hiking
- Jogging
- Shoveling
- Carrying heavy weights
- Cycling, greater effort
- Playing basketball
- Playing soccer
- Playing tennis (singles)

Figure 51

Being sufficiently active without engaging in regular physical exercise is almost impossible. In practice, the amount of energy used during most daily physical activities is relatively low, far below that burned during moderate- to vigorous-intensity exercise (see box and Figure 51). For everyone who does not have a demanding job, it thus becomes imperative to practice an activity regularly, like fast walking (by adopting a dog, for example), jogging or recreational sports such as badminton and tennis.

However, as we have seen, exercise alone is not sufficient to get the full preventive potential of physical activity if the time spent on it is negligible in relation to the total of all sedentary activities. It's absolutely necessary to find a way to use the 15 or so hours that remain at our disposal to be more physically active, even if only by avoiding sitting for long periods as much as possible.

What an active lifestyle might look like — combining moderate- to vigorous-intensity physical activity with very little inactive time — can be concretely illustrated by comparing the typical days of four office workers (Figure 52). The most sedentary person is obviously the one with the highest cancer risk: his day, totally lacking in physical activity, consists only of driving to work, sitting in front of a computer for 8 hours, and then going home, where he spends the remainder of the day

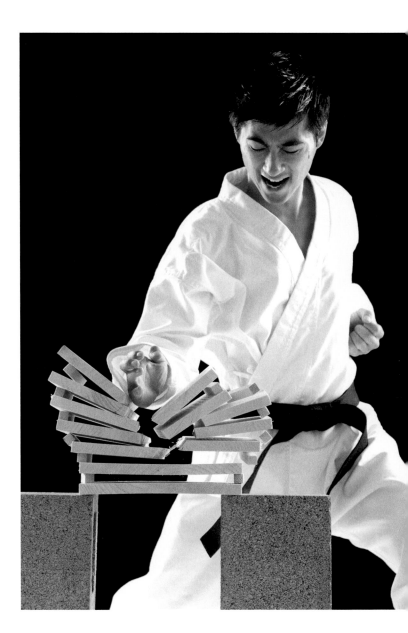

doing light tasks and relaxing in front of the television. The other three people are more active, each of them doing the same amount of average physical activity, but they will have different cancer risks depending on how they spend the rest of their time.

People who find ways to remain active all day long will get the most protection against cancer. Whatever works: stand up to talk on the phone (just standing up requires muscle contractions and burns three times the calories of sitting), take a break every hour to get a

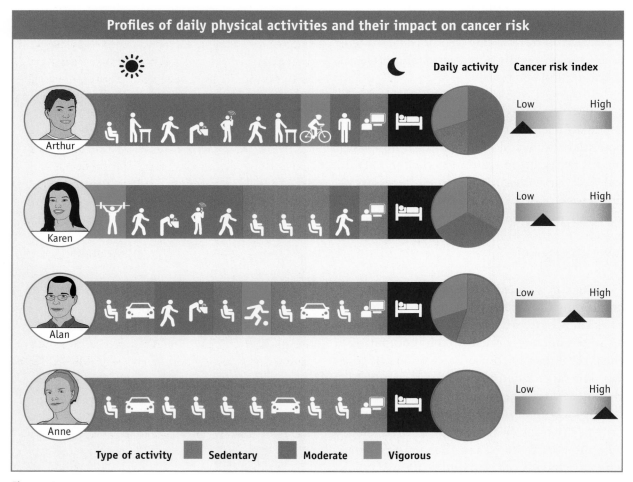

Profiles of daily physical activities and their impact on cancer risk

Daily activity   Cancer risk index

Arthur   Low   High

Karen   Low   High

Alan   Low   High

Anne   Low   High

Type of activity   ■ Sedentary   ■ Moderate   ■ Vigorous

Figure 52

Adapted from www.aicr.org, 2011.

drink of water, go outside for a walk during lunch hour, keep light weights handy for when you have to read a document, etc. The most important thing is to realize that being sedentary is an abnormal behavior, completely

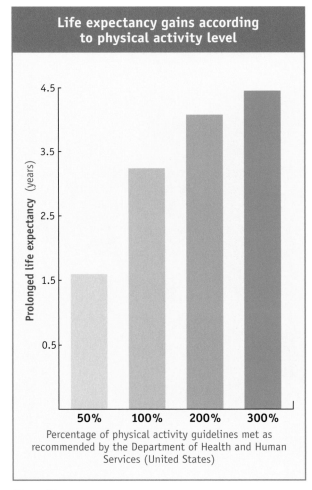

Life expectancy gains according to physical activity level

Prolonged life expectancy (years)

Percentage of physical activity guidelines met as recommended by the Department of Health and Human Services (United States)

Figure 53   Adapted from www.nih.gov, 2012.

unsuited to human physiology, and to avoid as much as possible remaining inactive for too long, whatever your activity is.

The increasingly sedentary nature of modern societies forces us, therefore, to redefine the role of physical activity in our lives. Currently, getting exercise is too often looked at only from the perspective of energy consumption, an activity whose only function is to burn calories to keep our figure or get rid of a few too many pounds. This narrow view can be dangerous, as it risks turning physical activity into a form of "punishment" that is only undertaken because we have to or to give ourselves a clear conscience. Yet the major positive effect of physical activity on the risk of developing some cancers and the disastrous impact of sedentariness on the incidence of the disease show the extent to which the benefits of an active life go beyond just maintaining normal body weight.

The many advantages of physical activity translate into a significant increase in life expectancy, with people who are the most active living on average more than 4 years longer than those who are sedentary (Figure 53). Along with quitting smoking, exercise may be the lifestyle change that will bring about the most health benefits, both for cancer prevention and chronic diseases in general.

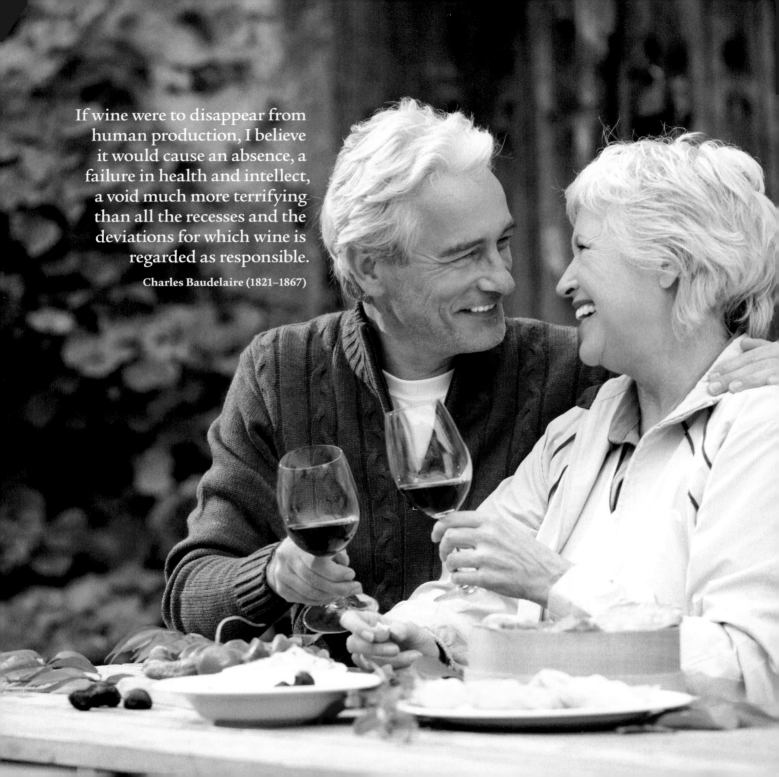

If wine were to disappear from human production, I believe it would cause an absence, a failure in health and intellect, a void much more terrifying than all the recesses and the deviations for which wine is regarded as responsible.

Charles Baudelaire (1821–1867)

Chapter 7

Alcohol, Red Wine and Cancer

Recommendation
Limit daily alcohol consumption to two glasses for men and one for women.

Source: American Cancer Society

Every night, an adorable Southeast Asian tree shrew, Low's ptilocercus (*Ptilocercus lowii*), spends several hours feeding on the nectar of palm tree flowers (*Eugeissona tristis*). At first glance, there is nothing surprising about this behavior, except that the nectar produced by this palm tree has the highest concentration of any natural alcohol source (3.8%), and the tree shrew consumes the equivalent of nine glasses of beer at each feed, yet shows no sign of drunkenness whatsoever! A tolerance to the alcohol naturally occurring in fruit has also been observed in some species of bat, which can "fly under the influence" without any difficulty, and in some insects like the fruit fly (*Drosophila*), which is especially attracted to very ripe fruit that may contain 1 to 2% alcohol.

Researchers have even shown that in these flies the brain's reward circuit is activated by alcohol, which leads males that have been sexually rejected by females to consume even more of this substance, almost as if they were trying to "drink" to "drown their sorrows"! The ingestion of alcohol naturally found in fruit, nectars and other sources of sugar is thus an age-old phenomenon, probably as old as the origination of fermentation by yeasts approximately 80 million years ago.

This evolutionary adaptation to the alcohol found in nature has over time been transmitted to humans. In addition to the "alcoholic tree shrew," believed to be the common ancestor of all primates, recent studies indicate that some of the great apes acquired the ability to metabolize alcohol about 10 million years ago. This adaptation may have been a consequence of living at ground level, where fruit fallen from trees was an abundant source of food, and contained — as it ripened — alcohol produced by fermentation from the metabolic activity of yeasts. This increased metabolic ability was a definite evolutionary advantage, as it gave the monkeys access to additional calories. Orangutans, on the other hand, who remained tree-dwellers, do not produce enzymes for the digestion of alcohol.

Alcohol is therefore not just any drug, in that our attraction to it is not merely due to its psychoactive effects, but perhaps also to the fact that it has long been part of our diet. This familiarity with alcohol also explains why the production of alcoholic drinks, whether beer, wine or rice alcohol, is closely linked to the evolution of the earliest civilizations, and has since time immemorial played a significant dietary role, as well as a ceremonial and religious one.

To Your Good Health!

Despite the large place that alcohol has always occupied in humanity's daily life, this substance is far from being harmless and actually has a very complex influence on health. This complexity is clearly illustrated by a "J" curve showing the relationship between the amount of alcohol ingested and risk of premature death (Figure 54). A synthesis of studies carried out on more than one million people shows that consuming

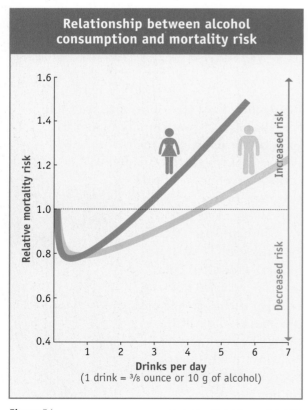

Figure 54   Adapted from Di Castelnuovo et al., 2006.

small amounts of alcohol daily (two glasses for men and one glass for women) is associated with a significant decrease (20%) in mortality risk, compared with people who do not drink, but that in larger amounts the protective effect of alcohol completely disappears and gives way to a large increase in risk of premature death, especially in women. According to the WHO, alcohol abuse is directly responsible for 3.3 million deaths each year, which corresponds to 6% of all deaths worldwide.

The protective effect of small amounts of alcohol is due in large part to a decrease in heart disease risk. Drinking one or two glasses of alcohol daily, of whatever kind, increases by about 10% the level of good HDL-cholesterol, which lowers the level of bad LDL cholesterol in the bloodstream and thus reduces the formation of atheromatous plaques that can cause coronary disease. Alcohol improves blood sugar control and has anticoagulant and anti-inflammatory properties, all factors that can contribute to a lower risk of heart disease.

However, the window of alcohol consumption that helps reduce mortality is much narrower than we might think. For example, daily consumption by a woman of more than $7/10$ ounce (20 g) of alcohol is enough to erase almost all of the positive effects associated with alcohol. For people who drink, this delicate balance means that it's important

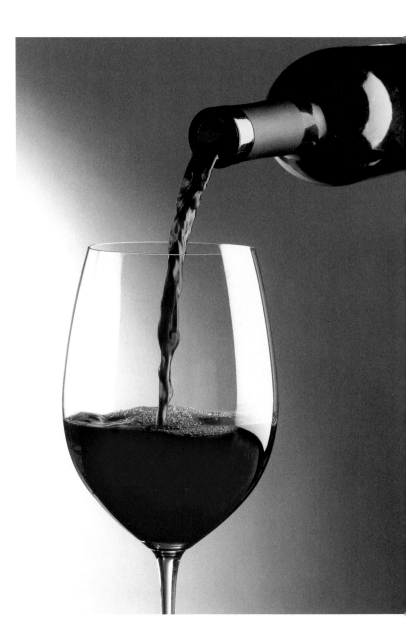

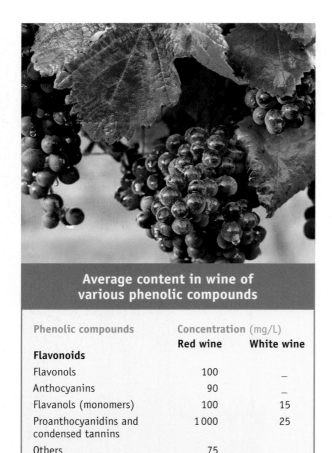

Average content in wine of various phenolic compounds

Phenolic compounds	Concentration (mg/L)	
	Red wine	White wine
Flavonoids		
Flavonols	100	–
Anthocyanins	90	–
Flavanols (monomers)	100	15
Proanthocyanidins and condensed tannins	1 000	25
Others	75	–
Nonflavonoids		
Stilbenes (resveratrol)	7	0,5
Benzoic acids	60	15
Hydroxycinnamates	60	130
Hydrolysable tannins (oak barrels)	250	100
Total	**1,742**	**285.5**

Figure 55   Adapted from Waterhouse, 2002.

to choose carefully the kind of alcohol with the most positive effects on mortality reduction.

Several studies indicate that regular moderate consumption of red wine could have benefits superior to those of other kinds of alcohol. A Danish study of 24,523 people showed that moderate red-wine drinkers have a risk of premature death three times lower than people who prefer beer or spirits (34% compared with 10%), an effect directly linked to the decreased incidence of heart disease and cancer. Similar results have been obtained in California and France and suggest that wine's unique phytochemical compound content, especially polyphenols, might in and of itself have positive effects that surpass those attributed to alcohol.

The Secret Lies in Fermentation

Wine is not an alcoholic drink like any other. Whereas beer and spirits contain only molecules with relatively simple and biologically inactive structures (carbonyls, esters, monocarboxylic acids, volatile acids), red wine on the other hand has several milligrams of phenolic molecules extracted from grape skins during the fermentation process (Figure 55). These complex molecules form part of a very sophisticated defense system developed by the vine to defend itself against ultraviolet rays

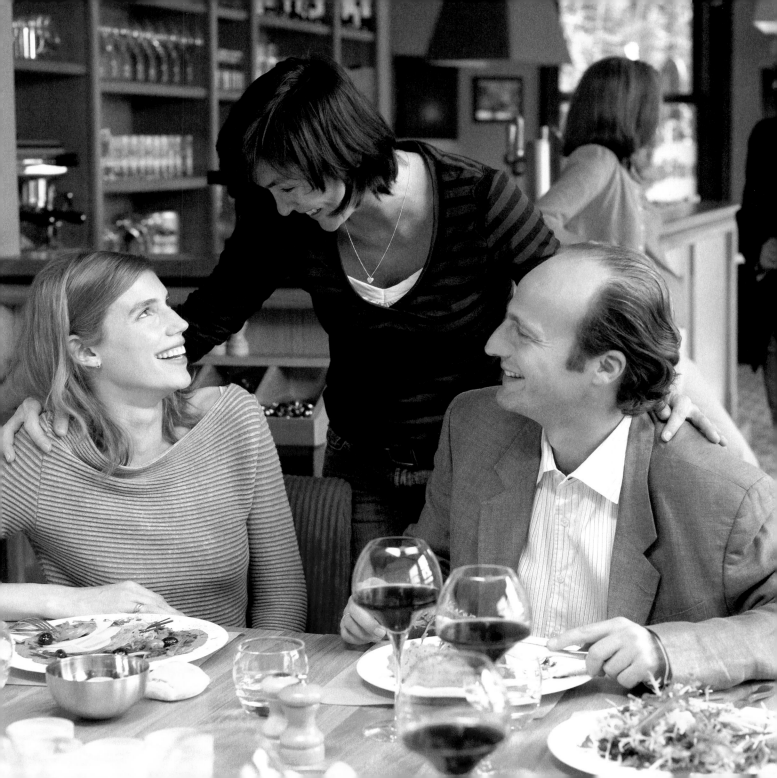

and various microorganisms that try to take advantage of the grapes' high sugar content. These phenolic compounds are absolutely vital to the organoleptic properties of red wine, and they also act in several ways on the human body, thus contributing to the positive effects of moderate consumption. White wines, fermented without grape skins, have a much lower quantity of these phenolic molecules and as a result have less pronounced beneficial effects.

Resveratrol is the molecule in red wine that has received the most attention to date, owing to its exceptional biological properties, especially its antioxidant, anti-inflammatory, antiplaque and vasodilatory action, as well as its many metabolic effects. However, proanthocyanidins and certain flavonols (quercetin) and flavanols (catechin) might also contribute to red wine's cardiovascular benefits. It's also interesting to note that red wine, even dealcoholized, improves blood vessel elasticity, increases plasma's antioxidant effect and decreases the oxidation of LDL cholesterol, parameters that are all associated with a cardioprotective effect. Because this positive impact is not observed after drinking white wine, which is largely lacking

< Resveratrol

in flavonoids and resveratrol, it's likely that the large amounts of phenolic compounds in red wine play a major role in the reduced risk of mortality observed.

Incomplete Detoxification

The beneficial effect of red wine on health must not make us forget that the alcohol it contains remains a very toxic substance that must be consumed with a great deal of moderation to minimize its harmful effects on health. Immediately after wine is ingested, the alcohol is absorbed by the stomach, and especially by the small intestine; it then makes its way very quickly into the bloodstream where it travels to the liver to be metabolized (Figure 56). Alcohol dehydrogenase (ADH) first oxidizes the alcohol into acetaldehyde, which is then transformed into acetate by aldehyde dehydrogenase (ALDH) in the mitochondria of liver cells. This metabolism is what changes a highly toxic substance (alcohol) into a harmless product (acetate), but this detoxification does not completely eliminate the alcohol's harmful effects, since the acetaldehyde formed during this reaction is a very reactive molecule that can cause enormous damage to cells' genetic material. Remember that acetaldehyde is related to formol (formaldehyde), which is usually used in pathology as a fixative for permanently preserving organic tissues ...

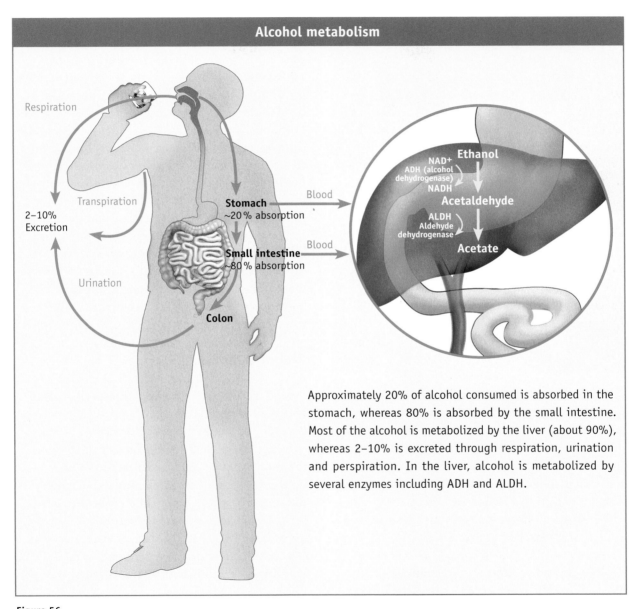

Alcohol metabolism

Respiration

Transpiration

2–10%
Excretion

Urination

Stomach
~20% absorption

Small intestine
~80% absorption

Colon

Blood

Blood

Ethanol

NAD+
ADH (alcohol
dehydrogenase)
NADH

Acetaldehyde

ALDH
Aldehyde
dehydrogenase

Acetate

Approximately 20% of alcohol consumed is absorbed in the stomach, whereas 80% is absorbed by the small intestine. Most of the alcohol is metabolized by the liver (about 90%), whereas 2–10% is excreted through respiration, urination and perspiration. In the liver, alcohol is metabolized by several enzymes including ADH and ALDH.

Figure 56

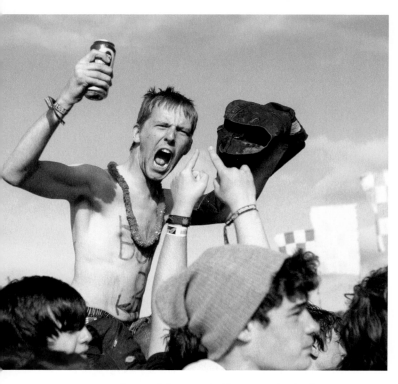

Several factors influence alcohol metabolism and are thus going to change the amounts of acetaldehyde generated during its digestion. In the first place, having food in the stomach slows down the absorption of alcohol somewhat. This is why it's always better to eat when consuming alcohol, especially for women, who are especially sensitive to its physiological effects (see box).

The rapid ingestion of large amounts of alcohol in a short period of time — the binge drinking especially popular among young people — is also associated with a very large increase in acetaldehyde. In addition to being harmful in the long term, these drinking sprees are dangerous in the short term, since they double the risk of stroke, even in young people. Differences in ADH and ALDH enzyme levels can also greatly influence a person's sensitivity to alcohol. Heavy drinkers, for example, have higher levels of ADH and can metabolize up to 1⅜ fluid ounces (40 mL) of alcohol an hour, three times more than a person who drinks reasonable amounts. Genetic variations can also influence the effectiveness of the ADH and ALDH enzymes, dramatically change alcohol metabolism and generate very significant amounts of acetaldehyde (see box p. 156).

Alcohol and Cancer

One of the best-documented effects of alcohol abuse is the increased risk of getting several cancers, especially those of the mouth, larynx, esophagus, colon, liver and breast. In 1997, the International Agency for Research on Cancer (IARC) classified alcohol as a Group 1 carcinogenic agent, a substance with proven cancer-causing properties in human beings. In most cases, however, the increase in cancer risk is not due to the alcohol itself, but instead to the acetaldehyde produced when it is metabolized.

Alcohol is Sexist

If a man and a woman of similar size drink the same alcoholic beverage, the physiological effects of the alcohol will usually be much more pronounced in the woman. This difference is explained in large part by the higher proportion of fat in the female body, which lowers the volume of water and immediately increases blood alcohol concentration. Women also have less alcohol dehydrogenase in the stomach, and this slower metabolism allows a greater quantity of alcohol to reach the bloodstream and come into contact with the body's organs. Women who drink large amounts of alcohol are therefore at greater risk than men of dying prematurely from the effects of diseases associated with excess alcohol, like cancers of the upper digestive system and breast.

Historically, alcohol consumption by women was a marginal phenomenon, and was even frowned upon, but major changes in the structure and functioning of modern societies have in most cases made these moral restrictions obsolete. In the West, for example, between 60% (United States) and 96% (Denmark) of women regularly drink alcohol, and sometimes in large amounts. In Canada, 20% of women go so far as to "binge" (four drinks or more in one evening) at least once a month, with this proportion going as high as 45% among women aged 18 to 24. Recent studies have shown that this high a level of alcohol consumption before a first pregnancy is potentially dangerous, since it considerably increases the risk of breast cancer. So we are not all equal in the eyes of alcohol, and women must keep in mind that they are physiologically more vulnerable to the harmful effects of this substance.

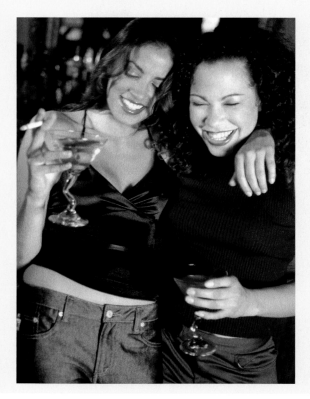

The upper digestive system (mouth, larynx, esophagus) is especially vulnerable to the effects of acetaldehyde. For example, just regularly using a mouthwash containing alcohol triples the cancer risk for these organs, apparently as a result of oral lesions coming into contact with the acetaldehyde formed by bacterial flora in the mouth. Drinking alcoholic beverages obviously poses an even greater risk, and Asians, whose alcohol metabolism has been altered by ADH and ALDH mutations, are up to 20 times more likely to get cancer of the esophagus, owing to the large quantities of acetaldehyde produced. This danger also threatens people with normal alcohol metabolism, but who drink large quantities of alcohol. Even the saliva of heavy drinkers contains an acetaldehyde level 10 to 20 times higher than that in their blood because of the transformation of alcohol into acetaldehyde by oral bacteria. This amount of toxic acetaldehyde can increase by 700% in people who smoke while drinking, a phenomenon that contributes to the powerful synergy between alcohol consumption and smoking in all of these cancers. For example, heavy drinkers (six or more alcoholic drinks a day) who smoke more than a pack of cigarettes a day are up to 40 times more likely to develop cancer of the oral cavity than those who drink moderately and don't smoke (Figure 57). The simultaneous use of alcohol and tobacco thus creates a particularly explosive carcinogenic "cocktail" that exposes the cells of the mouth, larynx and esophagus to very high concentrations of compounds that can damage DNA and trigger the emergence of cancer.

The amount of acetaldehyde that comes into contact with the organs of the upper digestive system can vary considerably depending on the kind of alcohol consumed. Some strong alcohols generate large quantities of this toxic molecule, even when they are ingested in small mouthfuls, not to mention that many of these beverages already contain acetaldehyde formed during their production (Figure 58). The worst example is without a

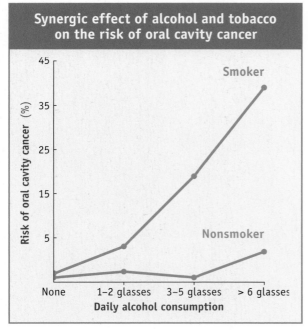

Figure 57 Adapted from Castellsagué et al., 2004.

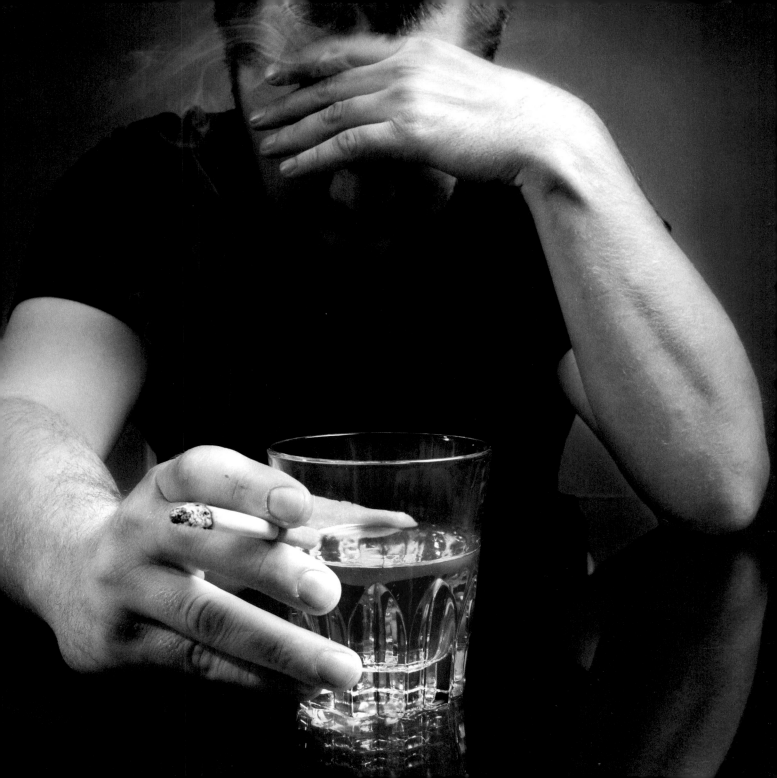

When Alcohol Makes Us Sick

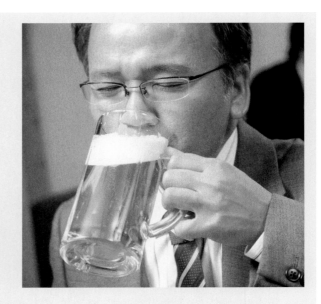

Many Asians, in particular those from Japan, Korea and China, have a "hyperactive" version of ADH (from 40 to 100 times more efficient than normal) that speeds up the transformation of alcohol into acetaldehyde. The rapid and sudden increase in the levels of this toxic molecule in the blood means that ingesting alcohol, even in small quantities, causes these people to experience side effects like rashes, headaches and nausea. This reaction, nicknamed the "Asian flush," is even more acute in people with another genetic defect, one that prevents ALDH from efficiently changing acetaldehyde into acetate. So much acetaldehyde accumulates following the ingestion of alcohol that it can cause tachycardia, violent nausea and vomiting. For the roughly 540 million people in the world who are deficient in ALDH, the severity of these side effects is such that total abstinence is usually called for.

Acetaldehyde content of various alcoholic beverages	
	Acetaldehyde concentration per drink (mg/15 mL alcohol)
Calvados	2.7
Other spirits (cognac, rum)	2.3
Beer and cider	2.7
Wine	1.3

Figure 58   Adapted from Linderborg et al.,2011.

doubt calvados, a cider brandy from Normandy whose consumption contributes to the very high incidence of esophageal cancer in this region of France. In contrast, it appears that red wine is much less damaging, not only because it contains half as much acetaldehyde as other forms of alcohol, but also because drinking it causes a much less pronounced increase in the salivary concentration of this toxic molecule than do beer or certain spirits. A study done on a million women indicates that although consuming alcohol other than wine increases the risk of mouth cancer by 38%, the increase is only 7% in moderate red wine drinkers.

It seems, therefore, that the greater decrease in mortality due to red wine consumption seen in several studies is linked not just to a more pronounced protective effect against heart disease, but also to a less harmful effect than other types of alcohol in terms of cancer risk.

Red Wine and Cancer

Red wine represents just 8% of alcohol consumption worldwide, far behind spirits (50%) and beer (35%). This is unfortunate, for not only does red wine seem to be less toxic than other alcoholic drinks, some research also suggests that this beverage may even have a preventive effect in relation to some kinds of cancer. For example, whereas beer and spirits drinkers are at a higher risk of getting lung cancer, moderate consumption of red wine, on the other hand, is associated with a significant decrease in risk for this cancer. In the same vein, the increase in risk for several types of cancer associated with alcohol consumption is not seen in red wine drinkers, with red wine even being associated with a decrease in risk for some cancers. These observations are consistent with the results of a large-scale study carried out on one million women over 10 years, showing that red wine might play a beneficial role in preventing several kinds of cancer (Figure 59). In some cases the protective effect seems mainly attributable to alcohol, with the consumption of any kind of alcoholic drink, whether red wine, beer or spirits, associated with a decrease in risk for four cancers, those of the thyroid, kidney and rectum, as well as non- Hodgkin lymphoma.

On the other hand, the increased risk of liver, mouth and colon cancer in beer and spirits drinkers almost completely disappears in those who prefer red wine, and the trend is even reversed in the case of colon cancer. Since these cancers are the collateral damage of regular alcohol consumption, these observations clearly illustrate the superiority of red wine and the importance of choosing this drink to get the benefits of alcohol while minimizing its negative effects.

In addition to their pharmacological action on heart health, polyphenols are also likely responsible for the positive impact of red wine on cancer risk.

Resveratrol, for example, is one of the plant world's most powerful anticancer agents, able to prevent cancer from appearing and discourage its development. In the laboratory,resveratrol inhibits the growth of a very wide variety of cells derived from human

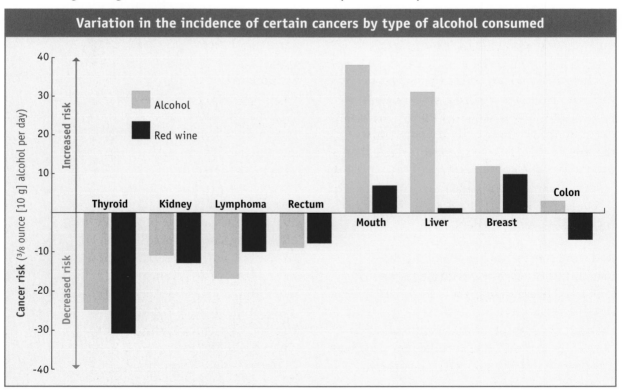

Figure 59

Adapted from Allen et al., 2009.

tumors by blocking their proliferation, or by causing their death through the apoptotic process. Anticancer activity is also suggested by resveratrol's ability to prevent the growth of several tumors in model systems. Resveratrol is metabolized very quickly after its intestinal absorption, however, and blood concentrations of the original molecule are relatively low, which raises doubts as to its actual ability to interfere with the development of cancer in humans. Recent observations indicate nonetheless that this metabolism does not seem to interfere with resveratrol's anticancer properties, as the molecule's metabolized forms, resveratrol sulfates, are captured by the cells, and resveratrol is then regenerated and can cause cancer cells to stop growing. Because of this mechanism, the concentrations of resveratrol absorbed through moderate consumption of red wine appear to be sufficient to interfere with cancer development, especially when these wines are made from grape varieties with considerable amounts of the molecule, in particular pinot noir (Figure 60).

Alcohol and Breast Health: An Impossible Marriage?

The link between alcohol consumption and cancer risk is more complex where breast cancer is concerned. Although a number of studies have observed a protective effect from red wine

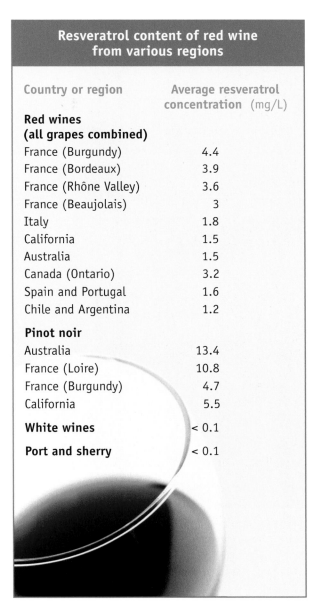

Resveratrol content of red wine from various regions	
Country or region	Average resveratrol concentration (mg/L)
Red wines (all grapes combined)	
France (Burgundy)	4.4
France (Bordeaux)	3.9
France (Rhône Valley)	3.6
France (Beaujolais)	3
Italy	1.8
California	1.5
Australia	1.5
Canada (Ontario)	3.2
Spain and Portugal	1.6
Chile and Argentina	1.2
Pinot noir	
Australia	13.4
France (Loire)	10.8
France (Burgundy)	4.7
California	5.5
White wines	< 0.1
Port and sherry	< 0.1

Figure 60   Adapted from Goldberg et al., 1995.

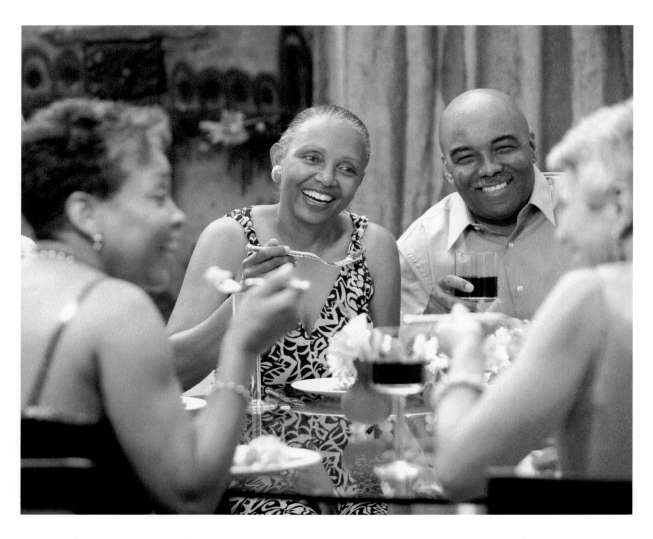

against the development of breast cancer, even in women at high risk because of a BRCA1 mutation, the moderate consumption of any kind of alcohol, including red wine, has been associated more than once with a slight increase (approximately 10%) in risk for this cancer (Figure 59). Given the high incidence of this cancer in the West, this observation is cause for legitimate concern. It's nonetheless important to remember that alcohol consumption is just one of many factors influencing breast cancer risk. Women who have never consumed alcohol in their lives, such as those living in some Muslim countries (Algeria, Pakistan, Egypt), have higher breast cancer rates than do Bolivian, Mexican or Polish women, who drink on average the equivalent of 8½ cups (2 liters) of pure alcohol a year.

The most important aspect of the health effects associated with moderate alcohol consumption in this age group remains the marked decrease in the risk of heart disease, which is much greater than the increase in breast cancer risk. For a 50-year-old woman, the risk of getting breast cancer in the next 10 years is 2.4%. An increase of 10% due to alcohol consumption brings this risk up to 2.6%, which translates into four extra cases of breast cancer per 1,000 women (Figure 61).

On the other hand, women aged 50 are at higher risk (46%) of developing heart disease, and the moderate consumption of alcohol lowers this risk by about 30%. In a population of 1,000 women, alcohol will thus result in 140 fewer cases of heart disease, a much greater benefit than avoiding the risk of four additional cases of cancer. In low doses, there is no doubt that the consumption of alcohol, and especially red wine, has an overall positive effect

corresponding to the decrease in mortality seen in epidemiological studies as a whole.

The complexity of alcohol's effects on human health is the best example of the caution that must be exercised in recommending or prohibiting certain habits to protect public health. Dogmatism and personal opinion are too often the rule when discussing these complex subjects, whereas what is important is to present all of the advantages and disadvantages of these habits and let individuals decide according to the health risk they feel able to handle.

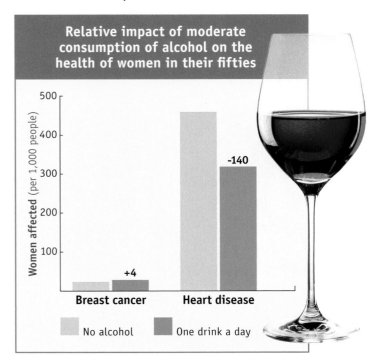

Relative impact of moderate consumption of alcohol on the health of women in their fifties

Women affected (per 1,000 people)

500
400
300
200
100

+4 Breast cancer

-140 Heart disease

■ No alcohol ■ One drink a day

Figure 61

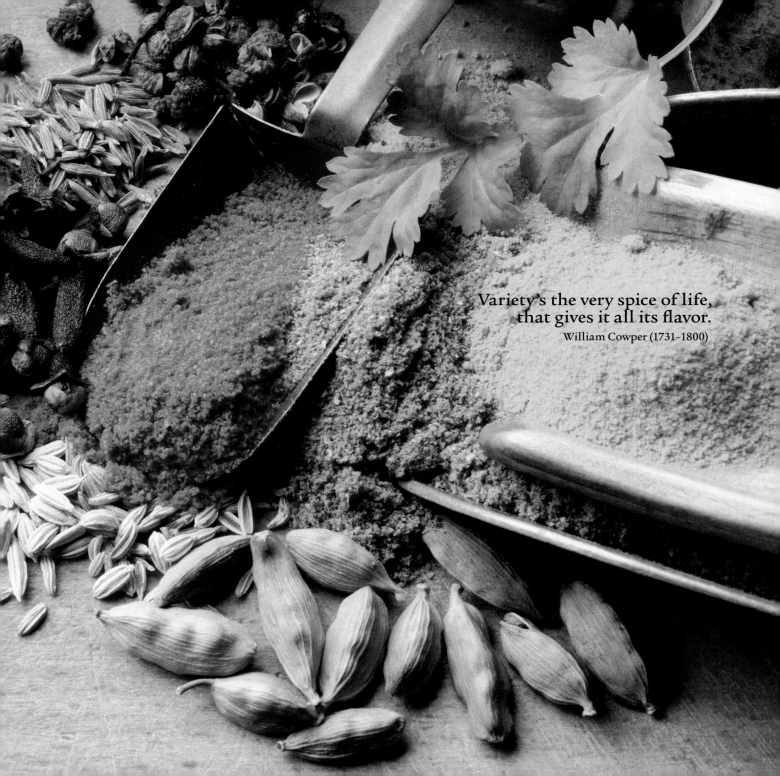

Variety's the very spice of life,
that gives it all its flavor.

William Cowper (1731–1800)

Chapter 8

A Salt-free Diet for Cancer Cells!

Recommendation
Limit consumption of products preserved with salt (salt fish, for example), as well as products containing large amounts of salt.

Source: World Cancer Research Fund International

Transforming food to make it more appealing is one of the acts that most sets us apart from other animals. It's the concrete expression of our desire not just to survive, but to live, to enjoy our brief existence to the fullest by seeking out pleasures that go far beyond the satisfaction of our basic needs. The conquest of salt and spices was thus a turning point in our history, not only because it completely changed our relationship with food, but also because it transformed the world we live in. For it was the attraction of salt and spices that lured explorers to the four corners of the earth and led to the discovery of new routes and new continents, and it is the trade in salt and spices that is responsible for the emergence of the colonialism and capitalism that reshaped the global geopolitical chessboard. Although these goods are now common and easily obtained food products, it must be remembered that seasoning a dish is not a trivial gesture, but instead a legacy of inestimable value from one of history's most important periods.

The Salt of the Earth

The salt we consume is one of the simplest minerals on the planet. It appeared over four billion years ago, when the water vapor formed by intense volcanic activity fell to earth as very acid rain, extracting the sodium plentiful in

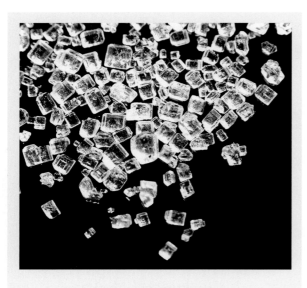

Salt or Sodium?

By far most of the sodium in our diet comes from salt (NaCl), and the terms sodium and salt are often considered to be synonyms. However, only the amount of sodium ingested matters from a health standpoint, and it's therefore the sodium content, not the salt content, that is indicated on nutritional labels.

Since salt is made up of 40% sodium and 60% chlorine, making the conversion is easy:
— to convert a quantity of sodium to a level of salt, multiply by 2.5;
— to convert a quantity of salt to a level of sodium, multiply by 0.4.

the earth's crust, combining with chlorine and accumulating in the oceans as sodium chloride or NaCl.

The first living organisms (archeobacteria) that appeared in these primitive oceans had to adapt to relatively large amounts of salt in their environment, so despite its apparent simplicity, this mineral played a very important role in the evolution of life. Even today, all living species need salt to survive, with some halophile (salt-loving) organisms having even retained the ability to grow in environments containing extreme quantities of salt, such as the Dead Sea (27% salt, compared to 3% for the oceans), or during the fermentation of certain very salty foods (soy sauce, fish sauce).

In human beings, sodium plays a critical role in the control of blood volume and pH, in muscle contraction and in nerve impulse transmission, and it's estimated that a minimal daily intake of about 500 mg of salt (200 mg of sodium) is required to make up for natural losses of the mineral, mainly through perspiration. For prehistoric people, products of hunting and gathering were the only source of sodium, and their salt intake was no doubt just high enough to meet their physiological needs. But the major dietary changes that accompanied the transition to agriculture — a lower meat intake and increased consumption of cereal plants containing very little salt

— threatened this balance and forced humans to put considerable effort into finding alternative sources of salt. The discovery that adding salt greatly increased the length of time foods could be preserved opened up a new chapter in the history of the human diet and turned this condiment into a substance indispensable to the survival of civilizations (see box on p. 166).

Salt and Cancer

Although preserving foods with salt made it possible to reduce fluctuations in seasonal availability, this practice had a negative impact on health. In addition to being closely associated with heightened blood pressure and increased stroke risk, salt is a major risk factor for stomach cancer, according to a great many studies. In North America, for example, stomach cancer was a significant cause of death at the beginning of the 20th century, but with the advent of refrigeration, fresh fruits and vegetables became more widely available and intake of salty foods decreased, leading to a dramatic drop in the incidence of this cancer. Similarly, several epidemiological studies have shown that high salt intake correlates with a marked increase in stomach cancer (Figure 62). The inhabitants of several Asian countries, for example, consume on average twice as much salt as Westerners and are especially vulnerable to this disease, with gastric cancer remaining

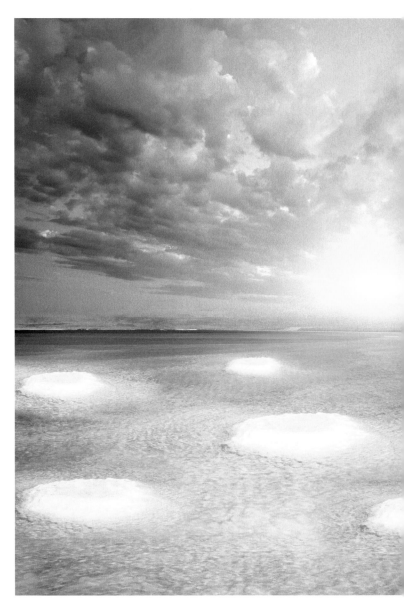

∧   Piles of salt in the Dead Sea.

165

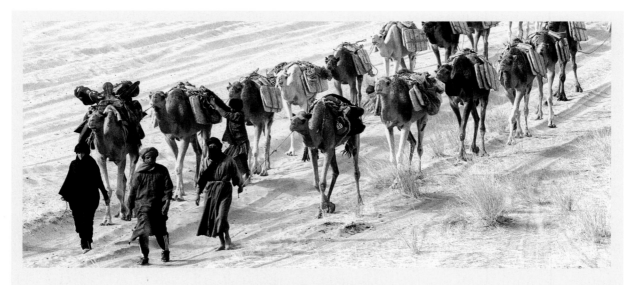

White Gold

Animals are instinctively attracted to salt, and watching them seek out salty terrain (salt licks), where they would lick the ground, likely gave humans the idea of using these salt sources to meet their own physiological needs. However, it was the discovery of its role in preserving foods that caused what can only be called a revolution in the use of salt. By dehydrating foods through osmosis, salt makes it possible to reduce contamination from microorganisms and considerably extend the length of time foods can be preserved, an especially useful property for populations traveling over large distances. As a result, salt quickly became an ingredient with great economic and political value, and the discovery of sources of salt and the control of roads used to transport it contributed greatly to the accumulation of wealth in a number of cities and states. For the Romans, for example, salt was indispensable to the expansion of the empire, and one of the first roads built was the *Via Salaria,* the salt road, linking Rome and the Adriatic. Roman soldiers were even paid with salt, a custom at the root of the word "salary," from the Latin *salarium* (salt ration). Most countries subsequently imitated the Romans and built roads for transporting salt; one of the most spectacular was that taken by the long camel caravans to cross the Sahara, which made Timbuktu in Mali the "pearl of the desert" in the 14th century.

one of the main tumors among the Japanese and Korean populations. This high incidence does not appear to be genetic in origin, as Japanese who immigrate to the West and reduce their salty food intake see a considerable decrease in their stomach cancer risk. Very salty foods are an important part of traditional Asian diets, including Korean *kimchi*, Japanese *miso* and *tsukemonos*, and Vietnamese *nuoc-mâm;* it seems that these food habits play an important role in the development of this cancer and also contribute to the high incidence in this region of nasopharyngeal cancer. It's interesting to note that countries where salt has played

a significant historical role — Mali with its African salt caravans, Chile with its large salt mines, or Portugal, where salt cod has long been an integral part of the diet — all have a high-salt diet that correlates with a high incidence of stomach cancer.

The Bacteria that Loved Salt

Infection from *Helicobacter pylori* is also known to be a major factor in stomach cancer risk. These extremely unusual bacteria are able to resist the highly acidic conditions in the human

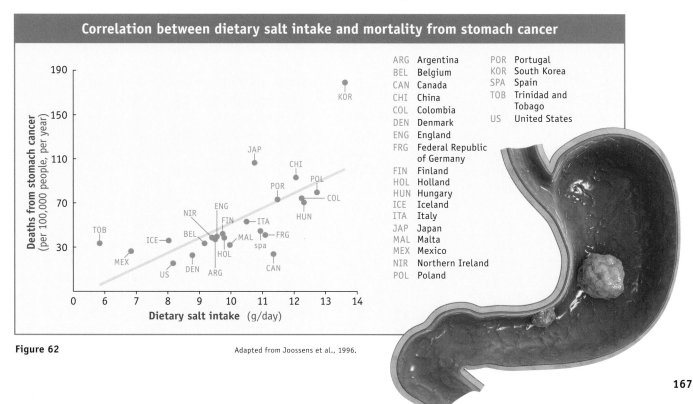

Correlation between dietary salt intake and mortality from stomach cancer

ARG	Argentina	POR	Portugal
BEL	Belgium	KOR	South Korea
CAN	Canada	SPA	Spain
CHI	China	TOB	Trinidad and Tobago
COL	Colombia	US	United States
DEN	Denmark		
ENG	England		
FRG	Federal Republic of Germany		
FIN	Finland		
HOL	Holland		
HUN	Hungary		
ICE	Iceland		
ITA	Italy		
JAP	Japan		
MAL	Malta		
MEX	Mexico		
NIR	Northern Ireland		
POL	Poland		

Figure 62   Adapted from Joossens et al., 1996.

stomach and can therefore successfully colonize gastric cells. Their propeller-shaped flagella (hence the name *Helicobacter*) enable them to "screw" themselves onto these cells, somewhat like a corkscrew — an adaptation that likely reflects the fact that we have lived alongside these bacteria for at least 60,000 years!

Half the world's population is estimated to be infected by *H. pylori,* but in most cases the infection is asymptomatic; in other words, the bacteria remain in a latent state without causing damage to the digestive system. In approximately 1% of infected people, however, the bacteria cause inflammation of the stomach lining, which introduces mutations into the cells' genetic material and increases the risk of cancer. Although these varying susceptibilities to the *H. pylori* infection may reflect the presence of distinct strains of the bacteria, recent studies suggest that too much salt in the diet could be what triggers this inflammatory cascade by stimulating the bacteria to produce precancerous proteins. In other words, without itself being a carcinogenic agent, salt can be considered a factor that promotes the onset and development of stomach cancer by providing *H. pylori* with the optimal conditions for expressing its inflammatory and oncogenic potential.

Plant Antibiotics

Eating large quantities of fruits and vegetables is associated with a decreased risk of stomach cancer that may in part be due to the ability of vitamin C to inhibit the formation of nitrosamines in the stomach and protect the cells of the lining from oxidative stress. It's also interesting to note that the phytochemical compounds in certain vegetables might help prevent stomach cancer by neutralizing the *H. pylori* infection. The sulforaphane in broccoli, for example, has a powerful antibiotic action against these bacteria, and a clinical study done in Japan has shown that eating broccoli shoots, an outstanding source of sulforaphane, cuts the levels of *H. pylori* in the stomach lining of infected people in half.

Salt in the Food Industry

Worldwide, salt has now become the main substance used to enhance the flavor of food, with each person consuming on average ⅜ ounce (10 g) of salt (⅐ ounce or 4 g of sodium) every day. Over 75% of this amount

< Electron microscopy of the *Helicobacter pylori* bacterium.

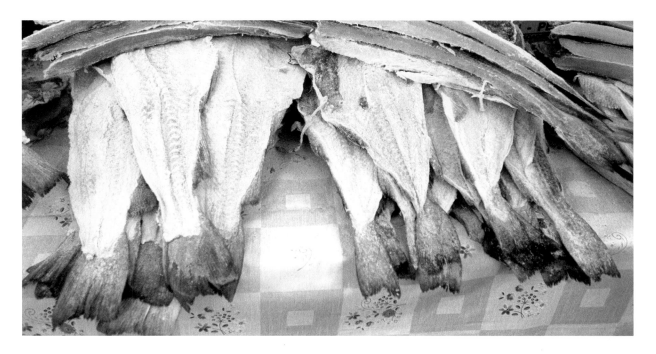

^ Salt cod in the Algarve, Portugal

comes from industrially produced food products and is thus eaten entirely involuntarily (Figure 63). This is too high an intake, almost three times the amount recommended by public health organizations (1/20 ounce or 1.5 g of sodium), and has harmful consequences for the body. It's estimated, for example, that more than 2 million people die prematurely from heart disease directly attributable to excessive sodium intake. Recent data have shown that salt in food can also accumulate in the body's tissues, where it activates certain immune cells known to play a part in the autoimmune system. The dramatic increase in autoimmune diseases observed over the past 50 years also coincides with the food industry's excessive use of this condiment.

Salt is part of our food culture and plays an essential role in the organoleptic properties of some dishes. For the food industry, on the other hand, salt is just a way to preserve or add a touch of flavor to mediocre-tasting products, exposing people to astronomical amounts of sodium, bearing no relation at all to the quantities our physiology is adapted to. The only effective way to decrease salt intake is to eat fewer of these industrial products and cook for ourselves as often as possible to "wean" ourselves off excess salt. And let's also remember that salt is not the only way to season a dish! There are several hundred different spices and flavorings from all parts of the world, and these delicious ingredients can lead us to explore new culinary horizons, not to mention that these plant products very often contain large amounts of molecules with many beneficial health effects, notably with regard to preventing cancer.

Spices for Good Health

The use of spices for culinary purposes is likely as old as humanity itself, with poppy, dill and coriander seeds having been found in sites occupied by prehistoric man more than 20,000 years ago. This taste for spices is especially well illustrated by the recent discovery of traces of garlic mustard seeds (*Alliaria petiolata*) in pottery used for cooking food approximately 6,000 years ago on the shores of the Baltic Sea. Since these seeds have very little nutritional value, but do have a peppery flavor similar to mustard, their presence attests to prehistoric cooks' early interest in spicy dishes.

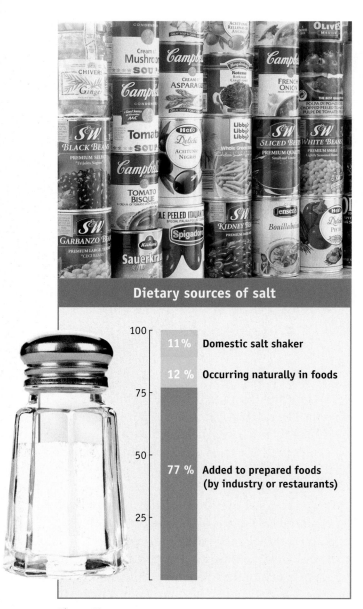

Dietary sources of salt

11 % **Domestic salt shaker**

12 % **Occurring naturally in foods**

77 % **Added to prepared foods (by industry or restaurants)**

Figure 63

170

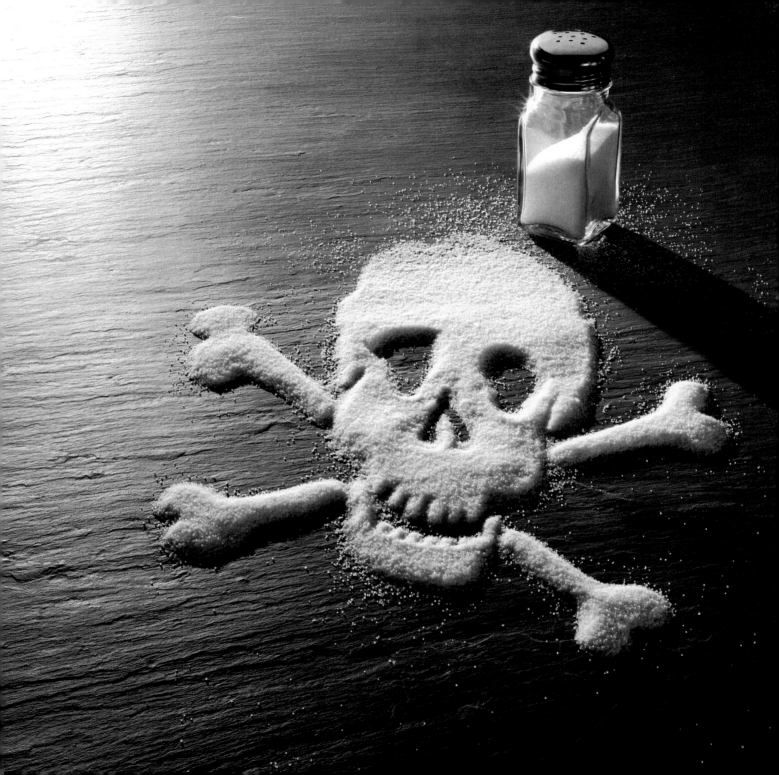

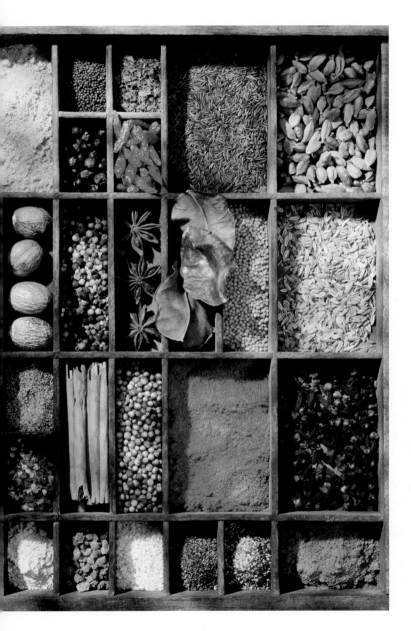

Several studies suggest that our attraction to spices stems not only from their taste, but in large part from their positive effects on health. Like all plants, spices and herbs produce large amounts of bactericidal, fungicidal and insecticidal compounds that are intended for self-defense, but that are also very useful in the human diet, since the antimicrobial action of spices and herbs makes it possible to preserve foods longer, especially meat. This is an especially important property for inhabitants of the hottest parts of the world: an analysis of the composition of meat recipes typical of these regions shows much larger amounts of spices than in dishes from Nordic countries (Figure 64). And these spices can sometimes be incredibly powerful, as gourmets who have experienced a particularly spicy South Indian *meen vevichathu,* Mexican *pollo mole poblano,* or Ethiopian *doro wat* can confirm! It's likely that people who frequently used these spices were in better health because they ate healthier foods, which helped spread this custom throughout the population as a whole, so that eventually eating very spicy dishes became a cultural characteristic common to several hot parts of the world.

Spices do not have to set your mouth on fire to slow down bacterial growth. Herbs like oregano, thyme, rosemary and coriander have antimicrobial activities that are every bit the equal of those of the pepper, chilies, nutmeg and turmeric of hot countries, with some extracts from these herbs even being active against the very dangerous meticillin-resistant *Staphylococcus aureus*. Although the first European contact with spices coming from India, Southeast Asia or Indonesia stirred up passions and acted as a catalyst for the exploration of the world, it was the bacterial properties of herbs growing plentifully around the Mediterranean basin that really played a leading role in the evolution of the culinary traditions of these regions, and these herbs remain today the "signature" of southern European and North-African cuisine.

Anticancer Spices

Spices and herbs are members of a select club of plants whose health benefits also include

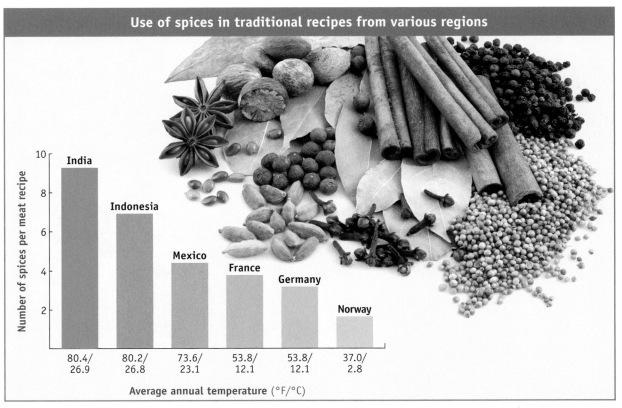

Use of spices in traditional recipes from various regions

Number of spices per meat recipe

| | India | Indonesia | Mexico | France | Germany | Norway |

Average annual temperature (°F/°C)

| 80.4/26.9 | 80.2/26.8 | 73.6/23.1 | 53.8/12.1 | 53.8/12.1 | 37.0/2.8 |

Figure 64

Adapted from Billing et Sherman, 1998.

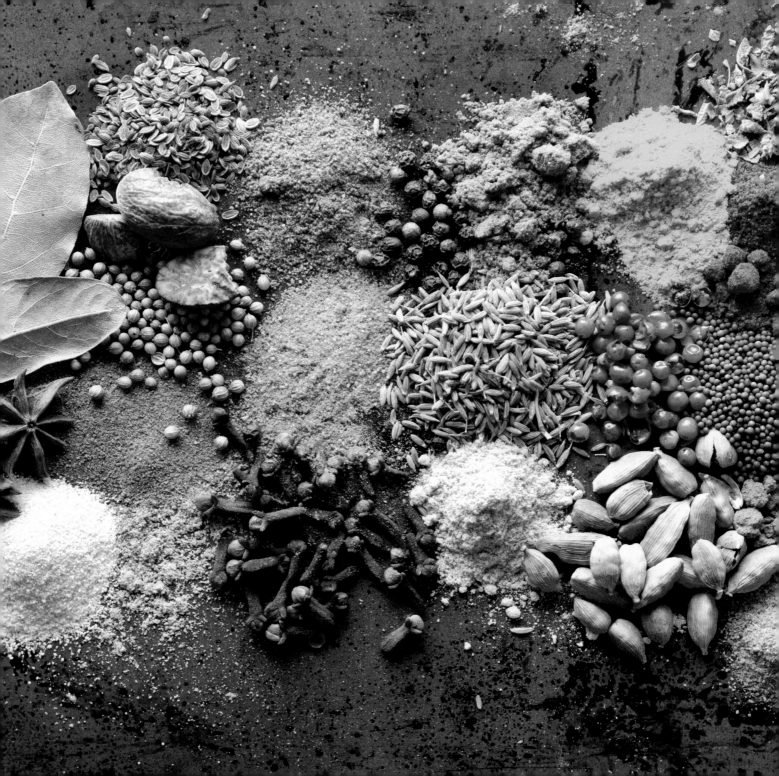

powerful anticancer activity. One of the first clues to this comes from observing that people who consume large quantities of spices, Indians for example, have an incidence of cancer four times lower overall than people living in countries with much less spicy food, such as Europe or North America (Figure 65). This difference is significant for several cancers that hit Western populations hard, colon and prostate cancer especially, with the incidence of these cancers being respectively 10 and 25 times lower in India than in the West. The consumption of spices is not, of course, the only factor responsible for these differences; cancer is a complex and multifactorial disease strongly influenced by lifestyle, and no single food, whatever its anticancer molecule content, can prevent the disease from appearing. Nonetheless, certain spices might play an important role in preventing cancer because of their high levels of polyvalent phytochemical compounds that can interfere in a wide range of processes essential for tumor development (Figure 66). For example, most spices have a strong anti-inflammatory effect that changes the cancer cells' environment, depriving them of the precancerous factors secreted by the inflammatory cells necessary for their growth. Some phytochemical compounds in spices and herbs can also block tumor growth by acting

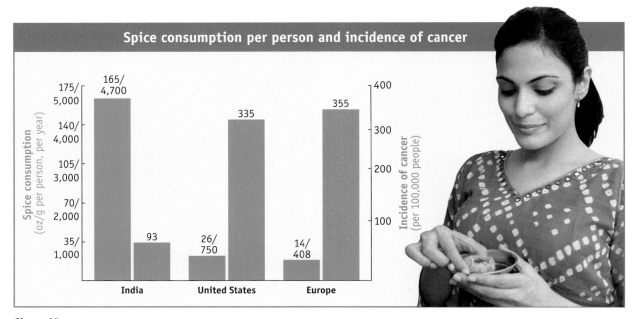

Spice consumption per person and incidence of cancer

Spice consumption (oz/g per person, per year)

Incidence of cancer (per 100,000 people)

India: 165/4,700 — 93
United States: 26/750 — 335
Europe: 14/408 — 355

Figure 65

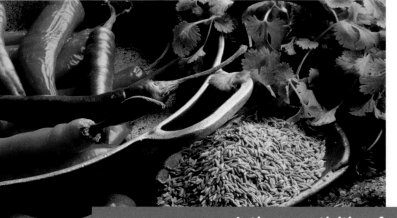

directly on cancer cells, either by stopping them from multiplying, or by causing them to die through the process of apoptosis

In some cases, the active molecules in spices and herbs can also stop the formation of a new blood vessel network through angiogenesis, thus "starving" cancer cells by keeping them from getting the nutrients and oxygen they need to survive. The culinary use of spices and herbs is, therefore, not just useful for adding

Anticancer activities of commonly consumed spices					
	Main active molecules	Anti-inflammatory activity	Inhibition of cancer cell growth	Apoptosis induction	Angiogenesis inhibition
Turmeric	Curcumin	•	•	•	•
Ginger	[6]-Gingerol	•		•	•
Chili pepper	Capsaicin	•	•	•	•
Cinnamon	Cinnamaldehyde	•	•		
Nutmeg	Eugenol	•	•		
Sesame	Sesamin		•		
Pepper	Piperine	•			
Parsley	Apigenin	•	•		•
Rosemary	Carnosol	•		•	
Coriander	Geraniol		•		
Basil	Ursolic acid	•	•	•	

Figure 66

Adapted from Aggarwal et al., 2009.

flavor to our daily dishes; these plants are concentrates of biologically active compounds with powerful anticancer activity and are able to slow down tumor cell development, thus preventing several kinds of cancer.

Turmeric, India's Gold

Turmeric is the best example of the benefits associated with a regular intake of these anticancer phytochemical compounds. It has been used for millennia by the peoples of India — traces of this spice have been discovered on the insides of cooking pots used 4,500 years ago by the Harappan civilization in the north-west of the country. Today, Indians alone consume 80% of the total world production of this spice, which translates into a daily food intake of about $1/14$ ounce (2 g) of turmeric per person.

Several thousand scientific articles published in recent years suggest that this high turmeric consumption might play a significant role in India's low incidence of several cancers. Turmeric is much more than a simple ingredient with a delicate flavor that blends beautifully with the more pronounced tastes and aromas of other spices, as in curries. It's a complex plant that contains some 235 distinct phytochemical compounds with anti-inflammatory and anticancer properties. However, it is turmeric's main polyphenol,

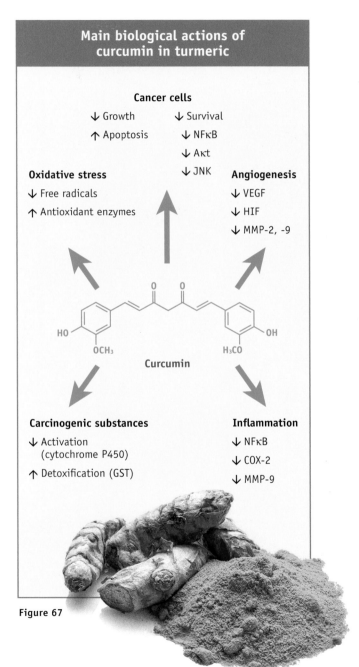

Main biological actions of curcumin in turmeric

Cancer cells
↓ Growth   ↓ Survival
↑ Apoptosis   ↓ NFκB
↓ Aκt
↓ JNK

Oxidative stress
↓ Free radicals
↑ Antioxidant enzymes

Angiogenesis
↓ VEGF
↓ HIF
↓ MMP-2, -9

Curcumin

Carcinogenic substances
↓ Activation (cytochrome P450)
↑ Detoxification (GST)

Inflammation
↓ NFκB
↓ COX-2
↓ MMP-9

Figure 67

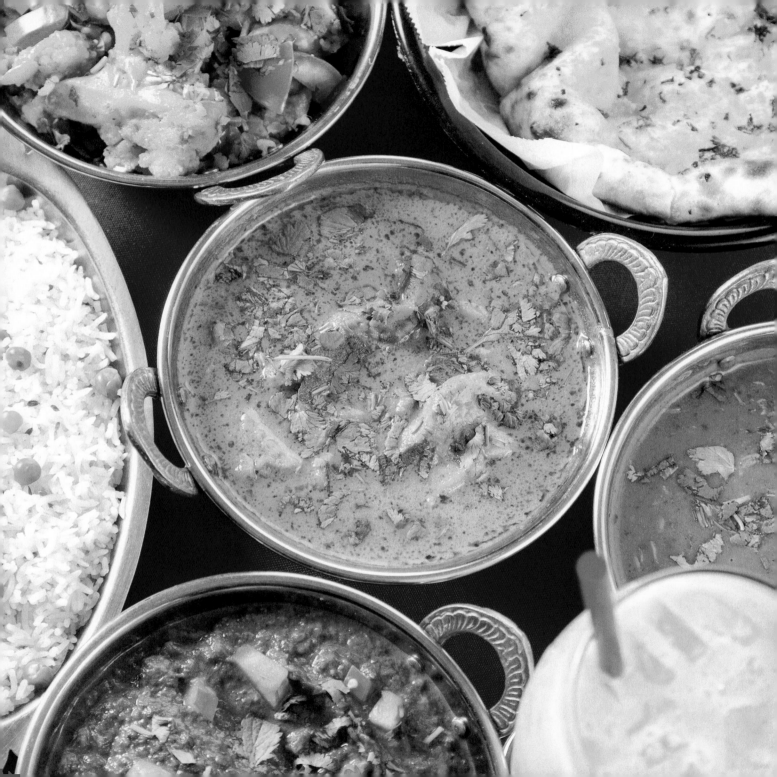

curcumin, that has received the most attention to date, owing to the large amount present in the spice (2–5% by weight), as well as its powerful inhibiting action on several processes involved in the initiation and progression of cancer (Figure 67). For example, curcumin is a first-line defense against cancer both because of its remarkable antioxidant activity, which protects against DNA damage caused by free radicals, and its effects on the metabolism of carcinogenic substances. By interacting directly with the body's detoxification systems, the spice prevents the activation of these carcinogens or speeds up their elimination from the body.

Several recent studies indicate that curcumin's outstanding anti-inflammatory action is the main reason for its beneficial effects on cancer. This molecule has the ability specifically to inhibit NFκB and COX-2 proteins, key regulators of the inflammatory response, and in so doing to reduce the production of factors that participate in the survival and development of cancer cells (see Chapter 1). Turmeric is thus one of the edible plants with the most powerful anticancer action, even raising the interesting possibility that this spice could be used for therapeutic purposes, for example as a complement to traditional radiotherapy. More than 60 clinical trials have been carried out, and 30 or so are currently underway, to measure the effectiveness of turmeric in treating various

cancers (colon, breast, pancreas, myeloma) and other diseases. The preliminary results are encouraging, since the consumption of turmeric and curcumin is well tolerated, even in relatively high doses, and some patients respond favorably to treatment. For example, one study suggests that curcumin enhances the response to chemotherapy in women with advanced forms of breast cancer.

Strength in Numbers

In addition to Asian and Indian recipes, turmeric can be added successfully to a wide variety of dishes, from soups to sauces to vinaigrettes. It has also become easier than it used to be to find the whole turmeric root, and using the spice freshly grated is an excellent way to enjoy its subtle taste; some studies also indicate that its antioxidant activity may be higher than in the ground spice. Curry powders on the market also contain turmeric, but the amount is five times less (0.3% compared to 1.5%, on average, for turmeric powder), so adding extra turmeric to these mixtures is a good idea.

Regardless of where the turmeric comes from, the golden rule for getting the most benefit from it is to increase its bioavailability by dissolving it in a fat with pepper. Curcumin is normally not well absorbed by the intestine,

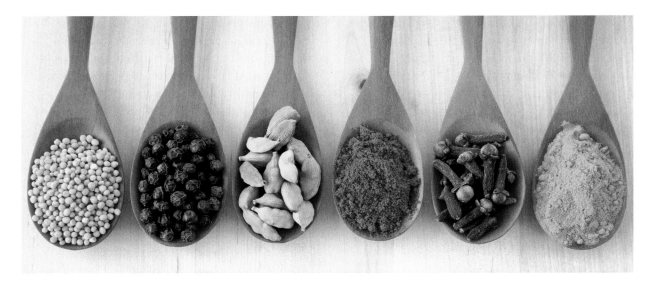

owing to its transformation by a class of enzymes called UDP-glucuronosyltransferases, but the piperine in pepper interferes with this metabolism and increases the absorption of the active molecule 2,000 times. Studies indicate that this piperine action is of critical importance if the curcumin is to counteract the damage done to DNA by carcinogenic agents and inhibit the growth of breast cancer stem cells. It appears that curcumin absorption can be greatly increased by adding other spices like ginger and cumin, two ingredients commonly used in preparing curries. This is yet another example of the great wisdom rooted in the world's culinary traditions, which have managed over time to identify the most effective combinations, in terms of both flavor and health.

A Gastronomic Experiment

Other spices and herbs also contain large quantities of phytochemical compounds and can contribute to preventing cancer. For example, apigenin and luteolin, two polyphenols especially plentiful in parsley and thyme, and the cinnamaldehyde in cinnamon, all have the ability to block the formation of new blood vessels by angiogenesis and could therefore prevent the onset of certain cancers. Anticancer effects have also been observed for the capsaicin in chili peppers and the gingerol in ginger. A diet including a wide variety of spices and herbs thus allows the absorption of an array of phytochemical molecules that, together, attack cancer cells on a number of fronts and can as a result have a synergistic impact that helps prevent cancer.

Nor must we ignore the major effect of spices on the organoleptic properties of the foods we eat, especially in an era when fat, sugar and salt saturate our senses and have become the main flavors we are exposed to. The monotony of this way of eating, in which satisfying our basic needs takes precedence over enjoying a range of flavors, can make us forget that eating is a unique sensory experience, the refinement of which has required millennia of experimentation in the world's varied culinary traditions. In some cases, the stimulation of the senses associated with the pronounced flavors of spices is quickly relayed to the brain and activates the satiety center, which means that people who eat spicy foods feel full faster and avoid absorbing too many calories. This anorexigenic effect is especially well documented in the case of chili peppers, with the decreased appetite associated with their consumption also being attributable to a decrease in ghrelin (the appetite hormone) caused by their main component, capsaicin.

There is thus no downside to using plenty of spices and herbs to season our daily dishes. They have no sugar or fat, and hence no calories, but, in addition, spices heighten our senses and allow us to create tastier and more satisfying food, while supplying the body with a number of plant molecules with anticancer properties. Recommending less salt in the diet is not just a good strategy for preventing heart disease and some kinds of cancer, it's the best way to spice up cancer prevention!

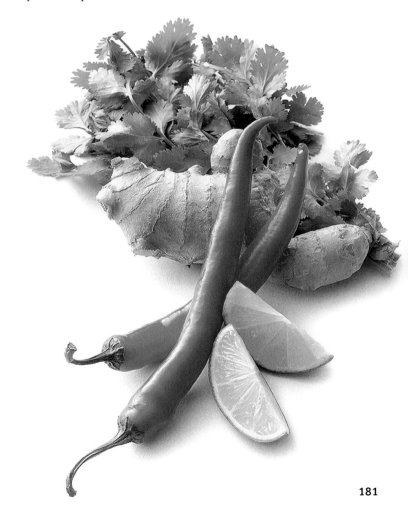

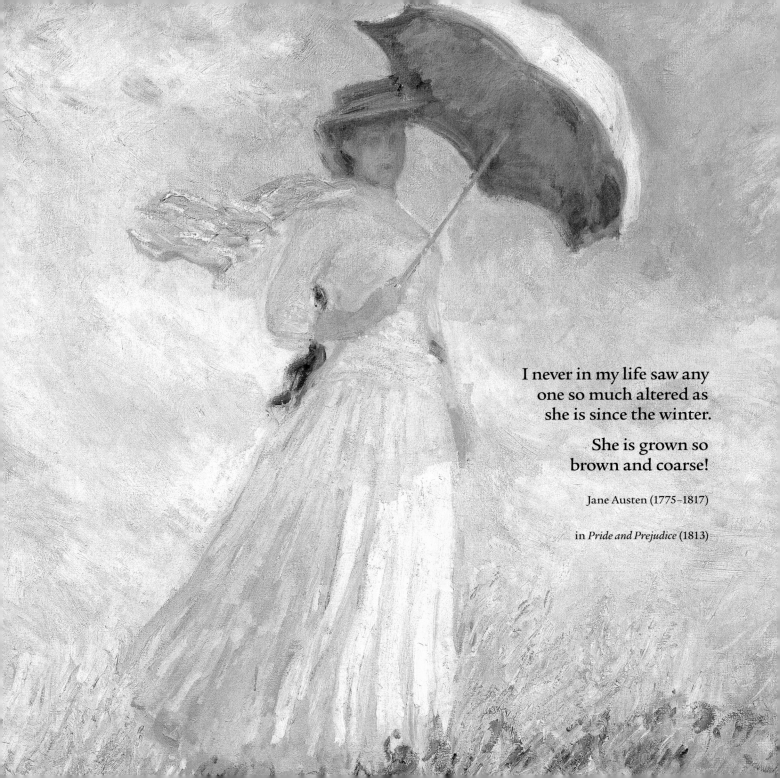

I never in my life saw any
one so much altered as
she is since the winter.

She is grown so
brown and coarse!

Jane Austen (1775–1817)

in *Pride and Prejudice* (1813)

Chapter 9

The Dark Side of the Sun

For most of the Christian era, a white face and skin has been considered a sign of superiority, both because pale coloring symbolized purity and the divine, and because it created a visible distinction between the elite and the common people, whose darker skin tone was a reminder that they were forced to work hard in the intense heat of the sun to survive. For the well-off, the sun was an enemy to avoid at all costs to protect their social reputation, a concern magnificently illustrated by the long garments, hats and parasols of people painted by many of the Impressionists of the 19th century. Pale skin was so important that it was sometimes accentuated with rice powder or even white lead-based makeup, despite the high risk of saturnism — lead poisoning caused by lead in cosmetics.

In a turnaround the secret of which is known only to history, the industrial revolution would completely change this attitude toward the sun. For with the migration of field workers into factories, workers were now the ones with pallid skin, which meant the upper middle class and the aristocracy had to rediscover the "virtues" of a tan to set themselves apart!

< *Woman with Parasol* (1886), by Claude Monet (1840–1926)

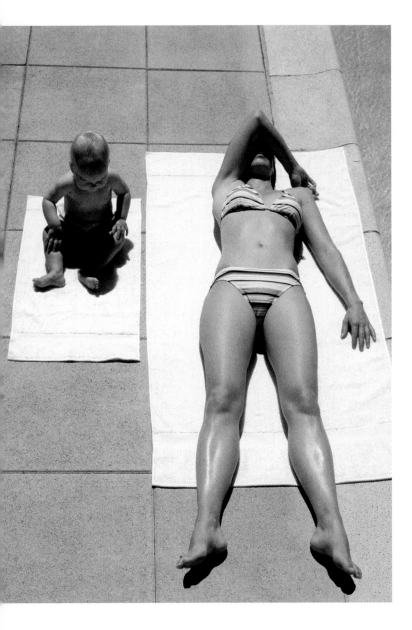

Fashion designer Coco Chanel is often credited with making suntanning popular, as she was one of the first prominent personalities to appear unashamedly with a suntan on her return from holidays on the French Riviera in 1923. But it was really the radical revolution in lifestyle that occurred at this time that acted as a catalyst, especially the new freedom in clothing accompanying the emancipation of women, who could now expose more of their skin, and the increased popularity of outdoor activities, made possible by paid holidays. Tanned skin became a sign of achievement and financial success, a luxury that showed you were different from ordinary people, who were slaves to their indoor work. In just a few years, a tanned skin went from being a sign of low social class to being a symbol of beauty and health, the visible expression of a dynamic and exciting way of life.

A Double-Edged Sword

As is often the case in life in general, neither of these extreme attitudes to the sun is entirely appropriate, with obsessive protection no more so than unlimited exposure. As early as ancient Greece it had already been noted that sun exposure could have therapeutic qualities, for treating tuberculosis and arthritis especially, knowledge that was used by the Romans in the invention of solariums (Aesculapius, the Roman

Rays and Radiation

Like all stars, the sun is a gigantic thermonuclear power plant that generates a phenomenal amount of energy through the fusion of hydrogen atoms. This energy is propelled toward Earth in the form of electromagnetic waves of varying lengths, consisting of 50% infrared (the source of the sun's heat), 40% visible light and 10% ultraviolet. All forms of radiation, whether radio, microwaves, visible light or gamma rays (radioactive), are caused by identical particles, photons, but they travel at different frequencies (Figure 68). A gamma ray photon emitted by a radioactive source, for example, travels at such high frequency that its energy can extract an electron from matter it encounters. This is called ionizing radiation. Ultraviolet (UV) rays have a lower frequency than gamma or x-rays and are called "nonionizing," but their energy is nonetheless high enough to damage biological systems by generating free radicals.

Since the bombs that struck Hiroshima and Nagasaki in 1945, everything "nuclear" has aroused great anxiety, but let's not forget that the sun's UV rays also result from the nuclear fusion process and that some of them can cause considerable skin damage.

As for the radio frequencies used by cell phones, some studies have raised the possibility of a slight increase in brain cancer risk (glioma and meningioma), which has led the IARC to classify this radiation as potentially carcinogenic (Group B carcinogens). Recent studies are reassuring, however, as they do not indicate a significant increase in brain cancer risk in the 10 years since cell phones were first used. Some studies have nonetheless reported a significant increase in neurinoma, a benign tumor of the acoustic nerve, in very frequent users. We cannot yet conclude therefore that there are absolutely no longer-term effects; as a result, several experts recommend limiting the length of calls, especially for young users, or wearing a headset instead of holding the phone to the ear. As for the radiation from cell towers, wireless internet access systems (Wi-Fi) or networked meters, this is much farther away from the body and studies done up to now indicate that it is not associated with increased cancer risk.

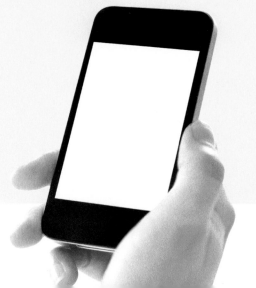

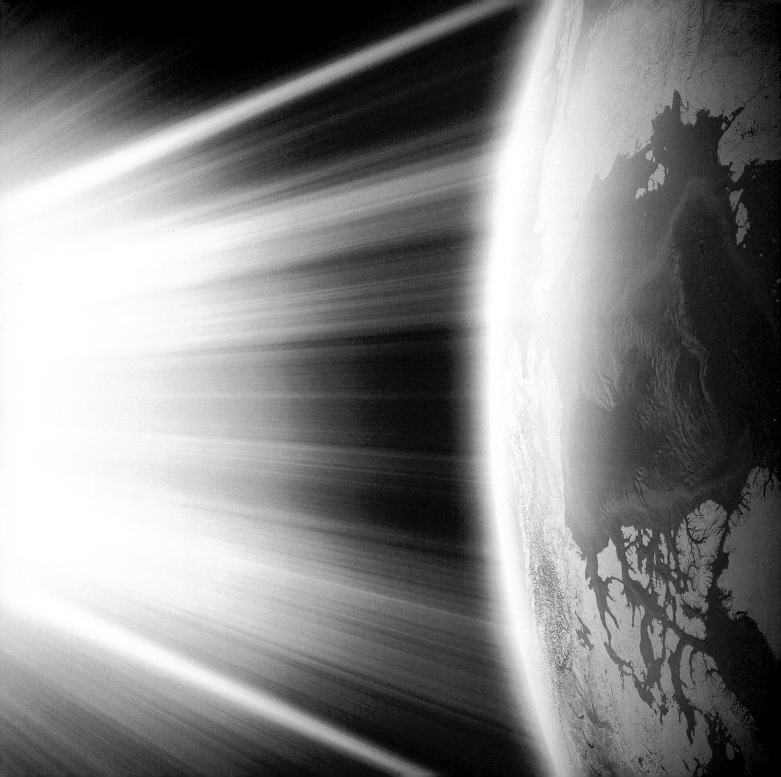

god of medicine, was the son of Apollo, the god of light). The great Persian doctor Avicenna was of the same opinion, but was nonetheless the first to note that too much sun was harmful and sunburn should be avoided. Even in ancient times, therefore, the sun was already known to be a double-edged sword — both too much and too little of it could be harmful.

We now know that the sun's dual action results from the wide range of electromagnetic waves in its rays, some of which have beneficial effects on health, whereas others can cause considerable damage (see box p. 185).

Significant Benefits

First, the positive: the sun is obviously essential to life! Visible sunlight makes plant photosynthesis possible, enables us to distinguish shapes and colors, and even,

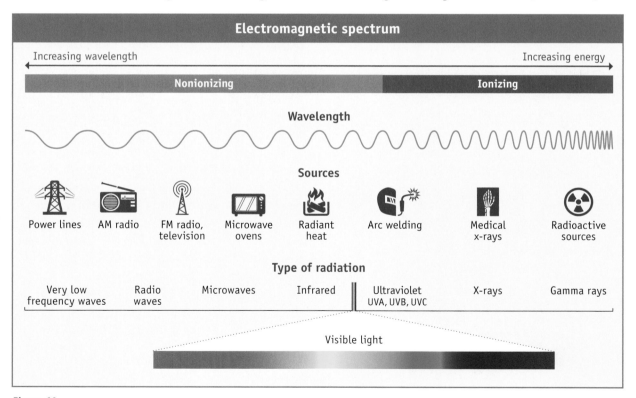

Figure 68

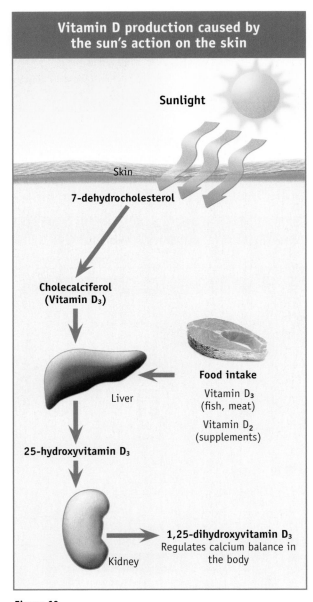

Vitamin D production caused by the sun's action on the skin

Sunlight

Skin

7-dehydrocholesterol

Cholecalciferol
(Vitamin D₃)

Liver

Food intake

Vitamin D₃
(fish, meat)

Vitamin D₂
(supplements)

25-hydroxyvitamin D₃

Kidney

1,25-dihydroxyvitamin D₃
Regulates calcium balance in the body

Figure 69

through our nycthemeral cycle, controls several of our physiological functions by means of the biological clock located in the brain in the suprachiasmatic nucleus of the hypothalamus.

The action of the sun's UVB rays on the skin also causes the transformation of a molecule called 7-dehydrocholesterol into vitamin D_3 (cholecalciferol), which is then changed by the liver and kidneys into 1,25-dihydroxyvitamin D, the biologically active form of the vitamin (Figure 69). Vitamin D plays a fundamental role in calcium and phosphorous absorption and is, as a result, a key bone mass regulator; in fact, a vitamin D deficiency in childhood causes rickets, a bone disease, which is why cow's milk is fortified with vitamin D in North America.

When it occurs over a short period of time, the effects of this radiation are limited to producing vitamin D; when the skin is exposed to the sun for too long, on the other hand, the extra energy it receives increases the likelihood that other cell components will be affected and damaged by the radiation. This is, in a nutshell, the crux of the problem surrounding the sun's impact on health: how can we enjoy the benefits of sun exposure while avoiding the problems caused by too much ultraviolet radiation?

Ultraviolent Ultraviolets

Ultraviolet rays are invisible and do not generate heat; they are emitted by the sun in three forms: UVA rays, by far the most plentiful; UVB rays, higher in energy but far fewer in number (5%); and UVC rays, very dangerous but completely absorbed by the ozone layer (Figure 70). Even though they are often considered less dangerous, given their lower energy, UVAs penetrate the skin more deeply and do significant damage by triggering the formation of free radicals that damage collagen fibers and cause the skin to age prematurely. The results of recent research indicate that the formation of free radicals by UVAs also contributes to the development of cancer.

UVBs are partially blocked by the ozone layer, but the rays that do manage to reach the earth's surface can cause a number of problems in the event of excessive exposure. Among these, the most common is the well-known sunburn, or erythema, which most vacationers experience, especially on trips to hot countries. Studies recently carried out have shown that this reaction is the visible (and painful) sign of a healing process triggered by healthy cells in response to damage caused by UVBs. The skin is "cleansed" of dead cells and those that have undergone genetic damage, by this physiologically beneficial inflammatory reaction. But this mechanism is not perfect

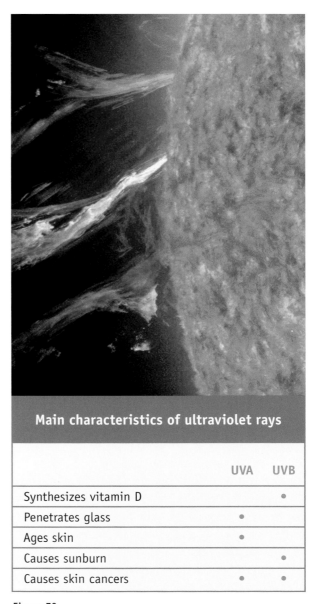

Main characteristics of ultraviolet rays

	UVA	UVB
Synthesizes vitamin D		•
Penetrates glass	•	
Ages skin	•	
Causes sunburn		•
Causes skin cancers	•	•

Figure 70

189

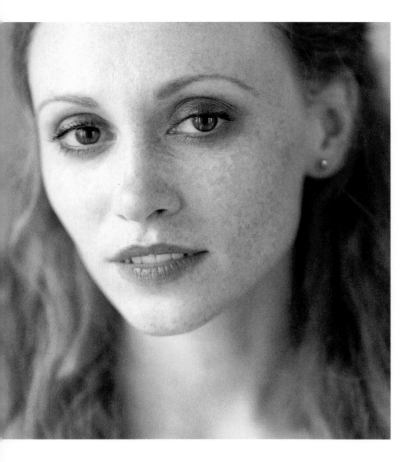

cancerous agents of the first order, able to cause the genetic mutations required for cancer cells to appear as well as to modify the cellular environment to foster their progression.

Pale Complexion

Melanin is the pigment chosen by evolution to protect the skin from UV rays, a property that stems from this complex polymer's ability to absorb radiation energy and thus reduce cell damage. Secreted by melanocytes in the epidermis, melanin has two distinct forms: eumelanin (black or dark brown) and pheomelanin (red or yellow). The difference in hair and skin color between one person and another is the result not of the quantity of melanocytes in their skin, but rather of the quantity and type of pigments they secrete.

The human species originally had black skin to protect it from the powerful radiation flooding the African continent. The migration of the first humans out of Africa was accompanied by major changes in pigmentation, especially in the inhabitants of colder countries. At these higher latitudes, a decrease in melanin and a whiter skin gave them a clear survival advantage, as the deeper penetration of the sun's rays into the epidermis allowed for increased vitamin D synthesis. This appears to be a relatively recent adaptation,

and repeated sunburns increase the risk that damaged cells will be unaffected by the "healing process" and become cancerous. Overexposure to these rays also causes the formation of free radicals as well as pathological inflammation, two processes that provide precancerous cells with an environment where they can develop. UV rays, whether type A or type B, are thus

however, as it's thought that the three genes responsible for fair skin only appeared in the European population 15,000 years ago.

These differences in skin pigmentation have major repercussions for people's sensitivity to prolonged UV exposure (Figure 71). There are six main types of skin, or phototypes, and the general rule is that the lighter a person's skin, hair and eyes, the higher the risk of skin cancer, up to 100 times higher than for someone with black skin. Redheads are especially at risk, as the pheomelanin they produce as the main pigment is not only less effective at blocking the sun's rays, but also generates large amounts of free radicals when stimulated by UV rays, which makes skin cell damage even worse. What's more, recent observations also suggest that redheads have an increased risk of melanoma, even in the absence of UV rays, owing to the oxidative stress caused by pheomelanin.

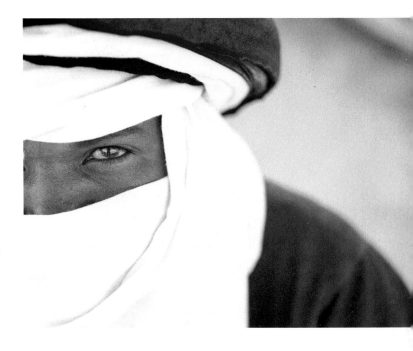

Although being born with dark skin is synonymous with a lower skin cancer risk, this does not mean that a person with fair skin can get the same level of protection by tanning. When the skin is exposed to UV rays, an important gene, the tumor suppressor p53, immediately detects the damage to cell DNA from the UV rays and reacts by orchestrating the production of melanin to protect the skin as much as possible from additional damage. This response is very important (most skin cancers are the result of a loss of p53) and is even associated with the parallel production of endorphins that makes sun exposure pleasant. But the protective power of this "emergency" melanin is limited and cannot prevent all of the damage caused by subsequent sun exposure. In other words, tanning is indeed the skin's defense mechanism, but it offers only very little protection, the equivalent of sunscreen protection factor 3. The situation is even worse for artificial tanning, since the UVA rays used in the booths provide no subsequent protection whatsoever from the sun's UVB rays, increasing cancer risk considerably (see box p. 196).

Fitzpatrick skin phototypes

	Type	Hair and skin color	Examples	Sensitivity to UV rays	Skin cancer risk
	1	Ivory white skin, very blonde or red hair	Scandinavians, Irish, Scottish (Celtic origin)	Extremely sensitive, always burns, never tans	Extremely high
	2	White skin, blonde hair	Caucasians from Northern Europe	Very sensitive, burns easily, tans minimally	Very high
	3	Medium white skin, chestnut/ dark blonde hair	Caucasians from Central Europe	Burns sometimes, tans gradually	High
	4	Olive skin, brown or black hair	Mediterranean and Hispanic individuals, some Asians	Burns rarely, tans easily	Low
	5	Brown skin, brown or black hair	Mediterranean and Middle-Eastern individuals, Indians, some African-Americans	Very rarely burns, tans profusely	Low
	6	Black skin, black hair	African-Americans, Africans	Never burns, tans profusely	Very low

Figure 71

Skin Cancers

Several studies conducted in recent decades have shown beyond any doubt that too much sun exposure equals a higher risk of skin cancer, including melanoma. After having evaluated all of the available studies on the topic, the International Agency for Research on Cancer (IARC) concluded in 1992 that UV rays were the main environmental factor responsible for skin cancer. The most common are basal cell carcinomas and squamous cell carcinomas, but melanoma remains the most dangerous, since it can enter the bloodstream and spread as metastases.

The main melanoma risk factor is intermittent and intense sun exposure, especially when accompanied by sunburn, whereas moderate and regular exposure has no negative impact and might even be associated with a slight decrease in risk. This increased melanoma risk is especially pronounced in people who are exposed to a great deal of sun in childhood, but still remains high for people who have had excessive exposure as adults.

The most worrisome aspect of melanoma is its sharp increase in recent years. Once very rare, the incidence of melanoma has gone up roughly 5% per year since the 1950s, the most dramatic growth rate of all cancers. For example, whereas an American's likelihood of

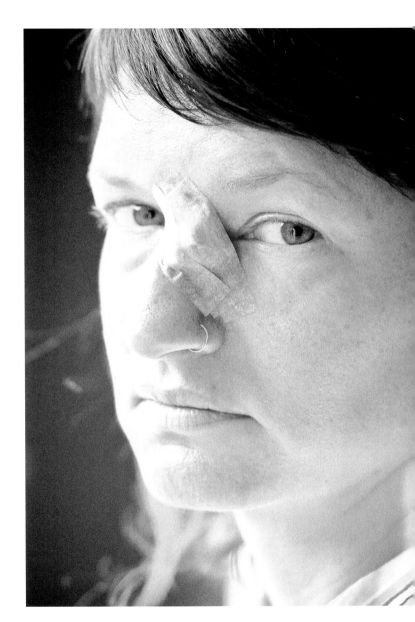

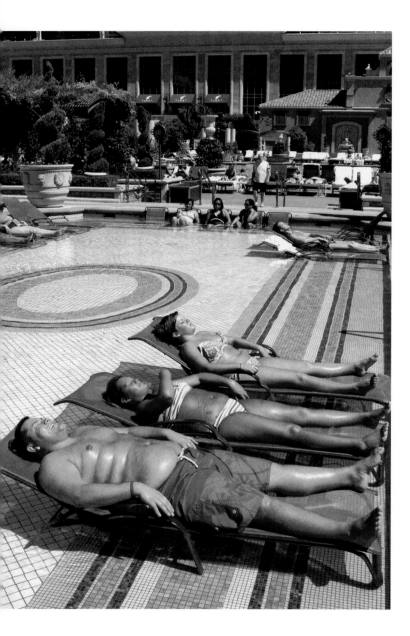

developing melanoma during his lifetime was approximately 0.07% in 1930, this risk had reached 2% in 2010, a nearly 30-fold increase (Figure 72).

By far the vast majority (85%) of people with melanoma are of Caucasian origin and live in wealthy countries. Oceania is the hardest hit, owing to its intense sunshine and significant proportion of fair-skinned people originally from northern regions. In 1999, people living in the Auckland area in New Zealand had the highest incidence of melanoma in the world. That said, melanoma, like skin cancers in general, also affects people living in less sunny countries. In Canada, for example, the incidence of skin cancer has exploded in the past 40 years, with the risk of getting a cutaneous carcinoma being three or four times higher and the incidence of melanoma 10 times higher (Figure 73). Even the Scandinavian countries, despite being located in the higher latitudes (>54° N latitude) and receiving 75% fewer UVB rays than countries on the equator, are hard hit by melanoma, with an incidence up to three times higher than sunnier regions like Italy and Spain.

Some of the increase in melanoma cases can be attributed to better detection, but these variations also reflect an important change in behavior with respect to the sun in recent decades. It's now common for people living in northern regions to regularly travel to warm countries in the winter, with the aim of getting a tan often being a major motivator to take one of these vacations. Since melanoma occurrence is directly related to occasional and intense sun exposure, these habits contribute to the increase in cancer in northern countries.

Sunscreen

The incorrect use of sunscreen is another factor that may contribute to the increase in skin cancer. Studies done on sun "worshippers" indicate that some people may use these lotions to increase the length of sun exposure and get an even darker tan. This behavior may explain why some epidemiological studies have uncovered an increased melanoma risk associated with sunscreen use, which led the IARC to conclude that these products encourage the development of melanoma if they are used during deliberate sun exposure. In other words, the amount of sunscreen applied and its sun protection factor are of very little value if the user's purpose is to get the darkest tan possible, since tanning indicates that DNA damage to the skin cells has already occurred.

Scientific research suggests, however, that applying sunscreen for preventive purposes reduces the risks of actinic keratosis (a precursor of skin cancer), squamous cancers

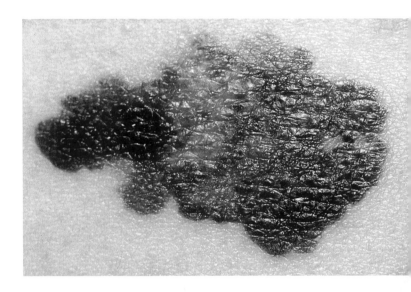

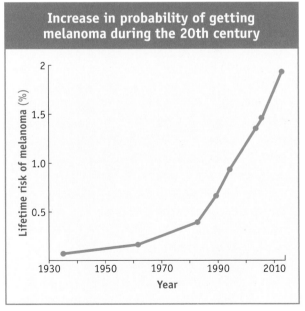

Figure 72 Adapted from D'Orazio et al., 2013.

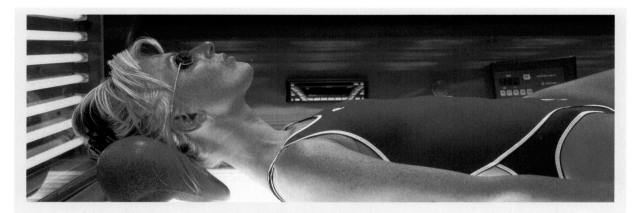

Canned Sun

A booming industry in North America and Europe, indoor tanning is advertised as a "healthy" alternative to the sun, a way to increase vitamin D levels without exposing oneself to the negative effects of sunlight. This is a strange idea, to say the least, in the sense that the UVA rays emitted by these machines are much less effective than UVBs for vitamin D synthesis. But the most dangerous side of these "canned rays" is their apparent cause-and-effect relationship, with a major increase in skin cancer — a 75% increase in melanoma risk — particularly in women. Furthermore, the International Agency for Research on Cancer (IARC) has recently included tanning beds in the highest category of cancer-causing agents, concluding that their carcinogenic potential is as great as cigarette smoke. Recent studies indicate that, far from being harmless, UVAs provide no protection from UVB rays, which means that people who get an artificial tan before their holidays in the hope of protecting themselves from the sun are exposing themselves to large doses of radiation with no idea of the danger involved. UVAs also trigger free radical production in the skin, an oxidative stress that can encourage the development of melanomas produced by the action of UVB rays. The melanocytes in fair-skinned people, which produce melanin in response to the sun, become vulnerable to UVA rays and can develop into melanoma as a result of the oxidative stress from the action of these rays. Indoor tanning must thus be avoided entirely, not just because of the false sense of protection artificial tanning provides, but especially because of the enormous risk caused by exposure to very high levels of carcinogenic UVA rays.

and melanomas in people who live in very sunny climates like Australia. The use of sunscreen with a sun protection factor of at least 15 is thus recommended for sun exposure lasting longer than 15 minutes. Recently, sunscreens that protect from both UVA and UVB rays have appeared, and these products are a very good choice for people whose activities involve spending long periods in the sun.

Melanoma Detection

Only recently have the dangers of UV rays been better understood, which means that most of today's adults were sunburned repeatedly during their childhood and are therefore more at risk of developing this cancer. It's therefore important to keep an eye out for skin melanomas, since when this cancer is diagnosed in its early stages it can usually be cured. Melanomas often resemble nevi, or moles, and sometimes develop from these spots. It's essential to pay close attention to the emergence of any nevi and to any changes in their appearance, especially if a close relative (mother, father, siblings, children) has already had melanoma. The so-called "ABCDE" of melanoma is an easy-to-remember guide (Figure 74).

It's also interesting to note that it was skin cancer that brought to light a surprising

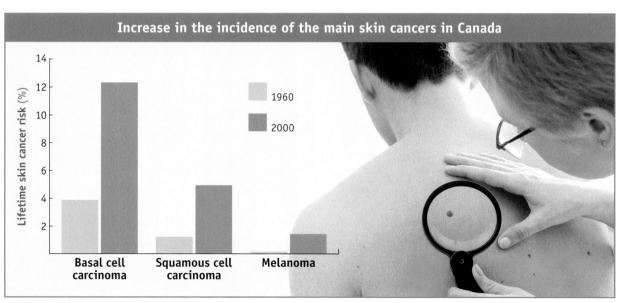

Increase in the incidence of the main skin cancers in Canada

Lifetime skin cancer risk (%)

1960
2000

Basal cell carcinoma · Squamous cell carcinoma · Melanoma

Figure 73

Adapted from Demers et al., 2005.

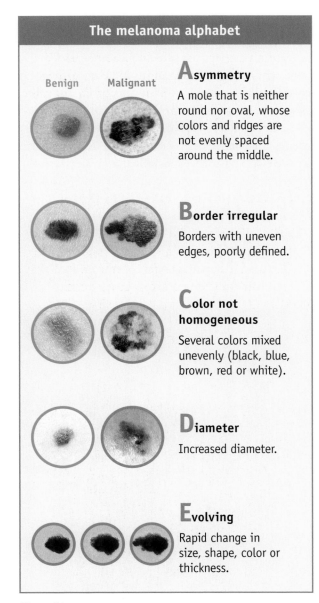

The melanoma alphabet

Benign   Malignant

Asymmetry

A mole that is neither round nor oval, whose colors and ridges are not evenly spaced around the middle.

Border irregular

Borders with uneven edges, poorly defined.

Color not homogeneous

Several colors mixed unevenly (black, blue, brown, red or white).

Diameter

Increased diameter.

Evolving

Rapid change in size, shape, color or thickness.

Figure 74

property of tumors: a specific smell, stemming from their unique metabolism and detectable by some dogs. These volatile metabolites are now being actively studied in a biochemical field called metabolomics (see box, p. 199).

It is sometimes said that the sun is "stronger" than it used to be and that this is why it has become so harmful. Obviously, this is not the case. The sun has been shining with the same intensity for billions of years; the reason skin cancer is increasing so dramatically is actually because our behaviors have changed, and people expose themselves from time to time to excessive amounts of ultraviolet rays. A small amount of UV is required by the body to stimulate vitamin D production, which plays a major role in calcium and phosphorous absorption from food and a key role in skeletal development, immune function and the prevention of certain cancers. There is no doubt that a little sunlight is good for health; however, just 5 to 15 minutes' occasional exposure of the hands, face and arms to the sun, two or three times a week in the summer, is more than enough to maintain this vitamin at optimum levels for health.

The sun must therefore be considered an outstanding source of a substance essential to health, vitamin D, but a source that is so powerful it must be treated with extreme caution. The sun must be respected and feared, not by totally avoiding it, but by exposing ourselves to the smallest possible dose, in order to enjoy its benefits while avoiding its dangerous side effects. We need to go outside to produce vitamin D, since UVB rays are absorbed by clothing and glass. The most important thing to remember is to avoid sunburn at all costs, as occasional and excessive exposure that burns the skin is the main risk factor for melanoma, especially when it occurs at a young age and in fair-skinned people. The vast majority of studies indicate that regular moderate sun exposure is not a significant risk factor for skin cancer, and might even reduce the incidence of some cancers.

The Smell of Cancer

In 1989, the medical journal *The Lancet* reported the strange case of a woman who had consulted a doctor because her Dalmatian would not stop sniffing a completely harmless-looking spot on her leg. A wise decision, as analysis showed the spot to be an extremely aggressive melanoma that would have left her with very little chance of survival if it had not been detected quickly. Several studies have since confirmed that dogs can detect a range of cancers, in particular breast, skin, colon and prostate cancers, sometimes even in the early stages of the disease. For example, some specially trained breeds (German shepherd, Labrador retriever) are able to identify 71% of people with lung cancer simply by sniffing their breath, and 97% of colon cancers when exposed to their stools. The abnormal metabolism of cancer cells seems to produce unusual volatile compounds that can be detected by dogs' very developed sense of smell.

Although systematic "canine screening" for cancer is not very likely, given the time it takes to train the animals, these feats indicate that cancer really does have a characteristic odor, and the development of cancer screening tests based on the detection of volatile compounds in patients' skin, breath, urine or stools may one day be possible.

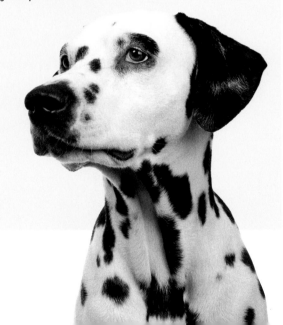

Happiness comes from the attention paid to small things, and unhappiness, from neglecting small things.

Chinese proverb

Chapter 10

Extra Protection

Not smoking, eating a healthy diet, watching body weight and getting physical activity can decrease the risk of cancer by two-thirds, and putting these lifestyle habits into practice is an essential part of any preventive approach. But in addition to these well-documented protective effects, research in recent years has also identified several other aspects of our daily lives that can influence in no small way our likelihood of getting cancer. It's well worth becoming familiar with these factors and the simple actions we can all take to maximize the likelihood of preventing this disease.

Recommendation
Young women should have themselves vaccinated against HPV.

Source: World Health Organization

< Particles formed from the capsid of the human papilloma virus (HPV), observed using colorized electron microscopy.

Worldwide, approximately 12% of all cancers are caused by infectious agents, a very large number of which are viral in origin (Figure 75).

Human papilloma virus (HPV) infections cause the majority of these cancers of viral origin and currently account for up to 5% of all cancers diagnosed every year worldwide. There are several dozen different HPVs, the most dangerous being the HPV 16 and HPV 18 strains, responsible for the vast majority of cervical cancers. Most women will be infected by one or another of these viruses during their lifetime, but the immune system will, in most cases, be able to neutralize them and prevent cancer from developing. When this defense fails, however, the incorporation of

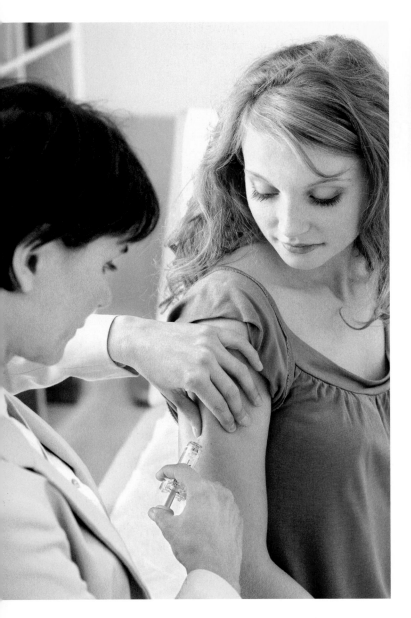

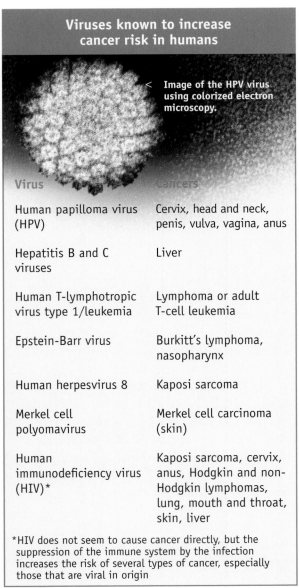

Viruses known to increase cancer risk in humans

< Image of the HPV virus using colorized electron microscopy.

Virus	Cancers
Human papilloma virus (HPV)	Cervix, head and neck, penis, vulva, vagina, anus
Hepatitis B and C viruses	Liver
Human T-lymphotropic virus type 1/leukemia	Lymphoma or adult T-cell leukemia
Epstein-Barr virus	Burkitt's lymphoma, nasopharynx
Human herpesvirus 8	Kaposi sarcoma
Merkel cell polyomavirus	Merkel cell carcinoma (skin)
Human immunodeficiency virus (HIV)*	Kaposi sarcoma, cervix, anus, Hodgkin and non-Hodgkin lymphomas, lung, mouth and throat, skin, liver

*HIV does not seem to cause cancer directly, but the suppression of the immune system by the infection increases the risk of several types of cancer, especially those that are viral in origin

Figure 75   Adapted from www.cancer.org, 2013.

viral DNA into the genetic material of healthy cells can result in the production of two proteins (called E6 and E7) that deactivate the functioning of two major tumor suppressors (p53 and Rb), causing the cells to multiply uncontrollably. A preventive approach thus remains key to fighting this cancer; as a result of cervical cancer screening with Papanicolaou tests (better known as Pap tests), followed by a colposcopy or biopsy for patients with precancerous lesions, the number of deaths from this cancer has been radically reduced in recent years, especially in the West.

However, the fight against HPV is far from won. The significant decrease in cervical cancer has been accompanied by a worrying increase in a number of cancers of the head and neck caused by this virus. For example, oropharyngeal cancer, which affects the part of the throat at the back of the mouth, including the base of the tongue, the soft palate and the tonsils, is 15 times more common in people infected with HPV. Historically, this cancer was a consequence of tobacco use, excessive alcohol consumption or a combination of these two factors, but with the decline in

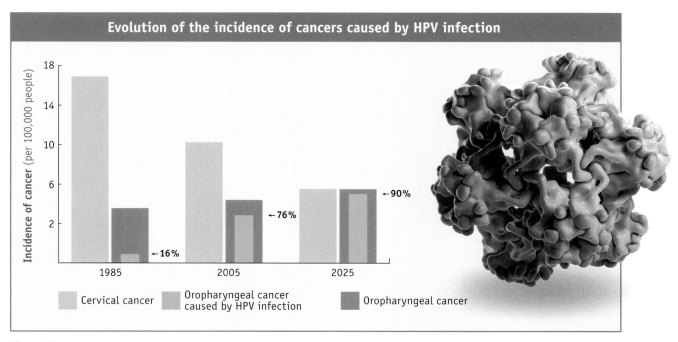

Evolution of the incidence of cancers caused by HPV infection

Incidence of cancer (per 100,000 people)

←16%
←76%
←90%

1985   2005   2025

Cervical cancer   Oropharyngeal cancer caused by HPV infection   Oropharyngeal cancer

Figure 76

Adapted from Chaturvedi et al., 2011.

smoking that has occurred in recent years, HPV infection has now become the main risk factor for oropharyngeal cancer. It's estimated that more than 70% of current cases are caused by the virus, a proportion that could rise as high as 90% in the coming decades (Figure 76). If this trend continues, specialists even predict that by 2020, the number of oropharyngeal cancers caused by HPV will exceed cervical and uterine cancers in industrialized countries. The increased incidence of oropharyngeal cancer could be the result of changes in sexual behaviors, since it's strongly associated with the practice of oral sex with a large number of partners. Recent studies indicate that the virus is found in the mouths of 7% of American teenagers and adults (10% for men and 3% for women) and could as a result be transmitted during this kind of sexual activity.

In recent years, vaccines that neutralize the action of HPV 16 and 18 have been approved for the prevention of cervical cancer, owing to their exceptionally effective action in hindering the development of precancerous lesions and genital warts caused by these viruses. Given the extraordinary results obtained to date, as well as the absence of major side effects, most public health agencies recommend giving these vaccines to young women before their eventual exposure to the viruses — in early adolescence, in other words. The recent increase in oropharyngeal cancers and the fact the virus

is found in the mouths of a significant number of men suggest that these vaccination programs should even be offered in the near future to the entire population, if the vaccines prove as effective in neutralizing oral HPV. Interestingly, a preliminary study indicates that one of these vaccines prevents 93% of oral infections from this virus. Meanwhile, limiting as much as possible the number of partners and using a condom are still the best ways to reduce the probability of contracting HPV or passing it on to one's partner.

Recommendation

Mothers should breastfeed their babies for a period of 6 months.

Source: World Cancer Research Fund International

According to the analysis done by the World Cancer Research Fund during the preparation of its second report, breastfeeding for a period of 6 months very slightly decreases (by about 2%) the risk of breast cancer in women. This effect likely occurs when gonadotropin production stops in response to prolactin secretion, since the resulting decrease in estrogen reduces the exposure of mammary tissue to these hormones. Recent data suggest that a similar effect might influence ovarian cancer, with women who have breastfed during their lives having a roughly 20% lower risk of getting this cancer.

Breastfeeding is of course beneficial for the child, but we too often ignore the impact of the mother's diet on the risk of diseases that their children may experience in adulthood. For example, women who adopt a diet mainly composed of high-sugar, high-fat processed foods expose their children very early on to these foods and can in so doing influence their food preferences for the rest of their lives. Studies suggest that exposing children to substances derived from junk food and present in breast milk can reprogram the brain's reward circuit and make them more dependent on the pleasure of sugar and fat, which can lead them to eat too much of these foods later on. High fat intake by breastfeeding mothers was enough to reprogram their babies' hypothalamus and disrupt their energy metabolism for their entire lives.

Breastfeeding is a very important period in the life of a mother and baby, not only because of the nutritional benefits of breast milk and the decrease in cancer risk for the mother, but also because it provides a unique opportunity to familiarize children with the taste of healthy foods, especially plants, and to influence their long-term health.

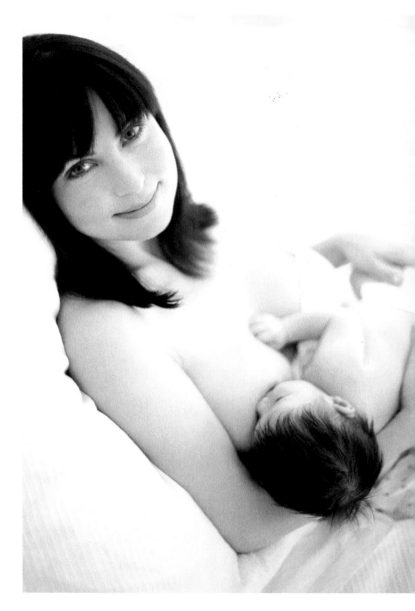

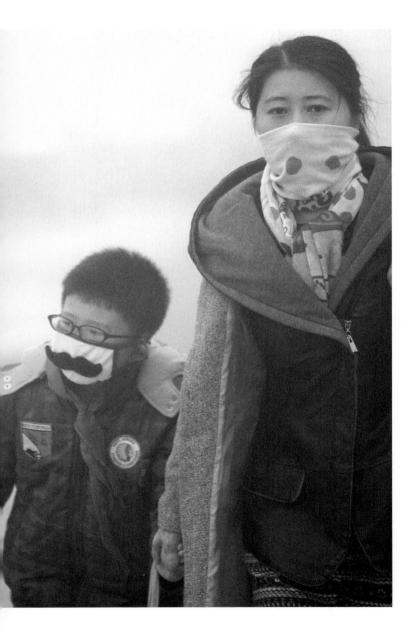

Recommendation
Exposure to chemical carcinogenic substances that cause environmental or indoor air pollution should be limited.
Source: World Health Organization

One of the most deplorable aspects of industrialization is the major environmental degradation that has accompanied the improvement in the standard of living of the population. Although we have the good fortune to enjoy unprecedented comfort and quality of life, the atmospheric pollution, global warming and toxic chemical residues that contaminate the water and soil are reminders that these advances have often been achieved at the expense of the welfare of the world around us, and that this situation can cause serious health problems.

Air pollution is the main source of exposure of the world's population to contaminants of human origin. According to the WHO's latest estimates, air pollution is responsible for approximately seven million deaths every year, with four million of these deaths due to indoor air pollution, while three million people die from the effects of exposure to outdoor air pollution. The vast majority of deaths (94%) are caused by heart and lung disease, with lung cancer responsible for just 6% of the deaths associated with this form of pollution.

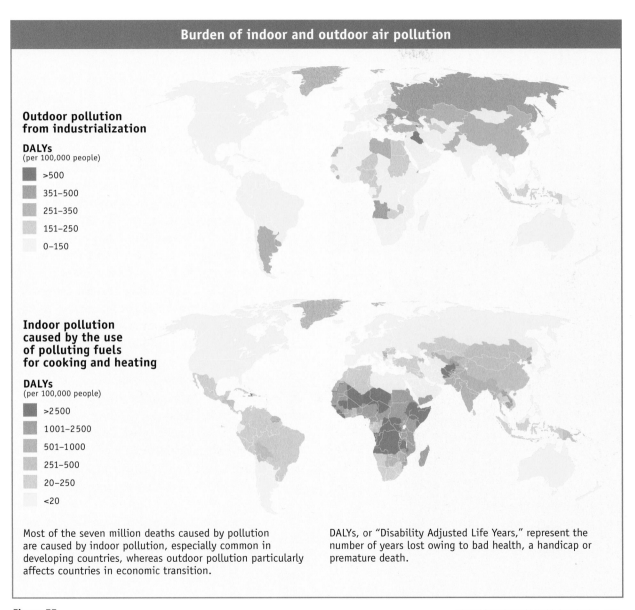

Burden of indoor and outdoor air pollution

Outdoor pollution from industrialization

DALYs
(per 100,000 people)

- >500
- 351–500
- 251–350
- 151–250
- 0–150

Indoor pollution caused by the use of polluting fuels for cooking and heating

DALYs
(per 100,000 people)

- >2500
- 1001–2500
- 501–1000
- 251–500
- 20–250
- <20

Most of the seven million deaths caused by pollution are caused by indoor pollution, especially common in developing countries, whereas outdoor pollution particularly affects countries in economic transition.

DALYs, or "Disability Adjusted Life Years," represent the number of years lost owing to bad health, a handicap or premature death.

Figure 77

Adapted from the World Health Organization, 2013..

The increase in lung cancer risk, caused by both indoor and outdoor air pollution, is a consequence of the carcinogenic effects of certain substances found in polluted air, especially diesel emissions, fine particles and some solvents. According to the WHO, these substances may be responsible for approximately 10% of the mortality linked to lung cancer, eight times less than cigarettes, but nonetheless a significant risk factor. Polluted air also appears to be associated with increased bladder cancer risk, a result of the process of eliminating these toxic substances through the urine and their interaction with the lining of this organ.

The burden imposed by air pollution is shared very unequally worldwide, however. Southeast Asia, regions in the western Pacific, and Africa are very hard hit by indoor air pollution, owing to the use of wood, coal or manure as the main sources of cooking fuel (Figure 77). The very rapid industrialization that has occurred in Asia in recent years has, on the other hand, contributed to the dangers associated with outdoor air pollution: roughly 85% of the three million or so deaths caused by air pollution in this region are the result. The residents of Hong Kong, for example, breathe air containing on average more than 30 µg of fine particles per cubic meter, or three times more than the WHO standard, whereas people in Ottawa, Canada, are exposed to just 5 µg/m³. However, the situation can be a great deal worse in a number of cities in China and India where levels above 200 µg/m³ have been measured.

This is an awful situation, since we cannot really control our exposure to these pollutants and eliminate the risks associated with them. Things must be kept in perspective, however: air pollution, however harmful, presents a much

Main risk factors responsible for diseases in North America, by order of importance (WHO)

1. Smoking
2. High body mass index
3. High blood pressure
4. Hyperglycemia
5. Physical inactivity
6. Diet low in fruits
7. Alcohol
8. Diet low in nuts and seeds
9. High cholesterol
10. Drugs
11. Diet high in sodium
12. Diet high in processed meat products
13. Diet low in vegetables
14. Air pollution
15. Diet high in trans fat

Figure 78   Adapted from Lim et al., 2012.

lower risk for cancer and chronic diseases than several aspects of our way of life, over which we have full control (Figure 78). In North America, the WHO estimates indicate that air pollution ranks 14th among the main risk factors for these diseases, far behind smoking, obesity, physical inactivity, alcohol and drug abuse and a poor diet.

Fortunately, society is becoming more and more aware of the damage associated with air pollutants, and standards aiming to regulate ozone and fine particles have been put in place in various parts of the world. In some regions, notably North America, the rates of contamination for several polluting substances have actually declined significantly in recent years. Much work remains to be done, though, and each of us can participate actively in resolving the problem by adopting a lifestyle that helps reduce atmospheric pollution. In fact, recent research suggests that foods with detoxifying properties, especially crucifers like broccoli, speed up the elimination of air contaminants and might thus be a first line of defense against damage caused by air pollution.

Environmental Toxins

In addition to air pollutants, many synthetic chemical substances are also found in water and soil, as well as in a number of commonly used products (insecticides, plastics, cosmetics, textiles) and even in our food (food additives, colorings, sweeteners). Their impact on health

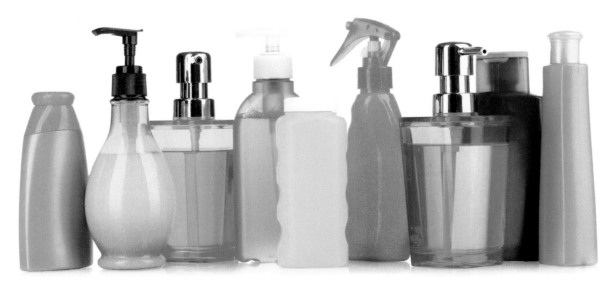

Main classes of endocrine disruptors	
Endocrine disruptors	**Main sources**
Bisphenol A	Plastics, resins, bottles, cans, dental amalgams.
Phthalates	Cosmetics, household products, PVC, packaging, toys, food packaging, solvents.
Parabens	Preservatives used in food, cosmetics, drugs.
Glycol ethers	Solvents, windshield washing fluids, deodorants, cologne, shampoo.
Polybromide compounds	Flame retardants (textiles, TVs, computers).
Perfluorate compounds	Stain- and waterproofing treatments (clothing, food packaging), nonstick coatings, waxes, insecticides.
Polychloride compounds (dioxins, BPC)	Incinerators, garbage dumps.
Pesticides (DDT, dieldrin, lindane, atrazine, trifluralin, permethrin)	Effluents on agricultural land.

Figure 79

has been the subject of a great many studies, but currently available data do not allow us to conclude that exposure to these molecules significantly increases cancer risk, at least in the quantities the majority of the population is exposed to. For example, large-scale studies clearly show that food additives, sweeteners like aspartame, and molecules like aluminum or parabens (used in deodorants, among other things) pose no health risk and do not increase the likelihood of getting cancer.

It is nonetheless important to emphasize that exposure to higher doses of certain environmental contaminants, particularly in the context of workplace exposure, has repeatedly been associated with increased risk for certain cancers. For example, several industrial chemical products have the common characteristic of acting as "endocrine disruptors"; that is, they can interfere with the normal functioning of the hormone system. These molecules are found in a wide range of industrial products (plastics, cosmetics, cans, household products and flame retardants, among others) (Figure 79), and can, in large doses, cause the development of various cancers of the reproductive system (vagina, breast, prostate and testicles). Studies have also reported that people who are exposed to relatively high doses of endocrine disruptors in the course of their professional activity may have an increased risk of getting certain cancers, notably breast cancer. It has also recently been suggested that toxic contaminants in some industrial products (gasoline, flame retardants, solvents, stain-proofed textiles) could increase the risk of breast cancer in women exposed to high doses of these substances, especially when this exposure takes place before a first pregnancy.

In our current state of knowledge, it therefore seems that the procancer effects of toxic substances in our environment are only observed in the presence of large quantities of these molecules, several times more than what the population is normally exposed to. The existence of an increased risk of cancer from higher doses of contaminants nonetheless indicates that we must remain very vigilant with regard to these substances and do everything possible to replace them with less toxic alternatives, or at least reduce their presence in the environment to a minimum. This distrust is all the more important since new synthetic molecules are constantly appearing in our daily lives, without their long-term impact on health being clearly established. Carbon nanotubes are a good example; these nanotechnology products are being used to make a growing number of products, both for industrial use (in the aerospace, electronics, automobile and medical industries) and for domestic use (in paints, sunscreens, cosmetics). Unfortunately, the marketing of these new products is poorly regulated, with few controls, and the safety of

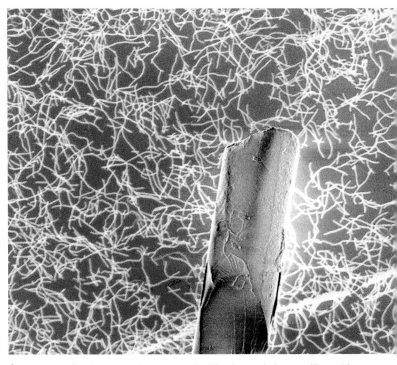

∧   Network of carbon nanotubes compared with a human hair on a silicon chip.

these new molecules is far from being proven. It must be remembered that nanomaterials are 50,000 times smaller than the thickness of a hair and can therefore pass through physiological barriers and accumulate in the tissues, where they can cause lesions. These particles are also very lightweight; they can thus be airborne and inhaled into the lungs, just like asbestos fibers. The impact of these nanoparticles on cancer risk remains to be established, but recent studies indicate that they might speed up the development of adenocarcinomas in the lungs of animals. These observations are worrying, given that nanotechnologies are booming, and the use of nanoparticles to administer certain drugs is even being envisaged. Just as with all the foreign substances we are exposed to, the precautionary principle should apply to nanoparticles, and a very rigorous evaluation of their impact on human health would be desirable before these substances become ubiquitous.

It is no doubt in our nature to cite the role of external factors beyond our control to explain the problems that affect us, but it's important to view the risks posed by these factors in relative terms and to remind ourselves that it is still first and foremost our lifestyle habits that play the largest role in the high incidence of cancer in industrialized countries.

Radon, a Radioactive Gas

Radon 222 (^{222}Rn) is an inert and odorless gas produced by the radioactive disintegration of the uranium occurring naturally in the earth's crust. This radioactive gas alone accounts for half the radiation from natural sources we are exposed to, an amount that is still lower, however, than that emitted by various modern medical techniques like imaging or radiotherapy (Figure 80). In addition, it's important to note that the radiation from a CT

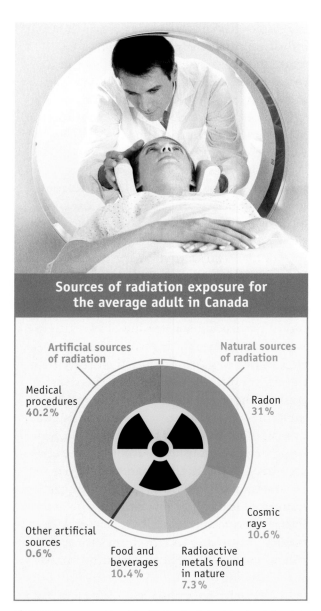

Sources of radiation exposure for the average adult in Canada

Artificial sources of radiation

Natural sources of radiation

Medical procedures 40.2%

Radon 31%

Other artificial sources 0.6%

Food and beverages 10.4%

Radioactive metals found in nature 7.3%

Cosmic rays 10.6%

Figure 80   Adapted from lthe Canadian Nuclear Safety Commission, 2012..

scan can be 1,000 times higher than radiation from traditional x-rays, which has experts worrying that the excessive use of this technique, as practiced in some countries, could cause an increase in cancers in the near future. As for radon, its concentrations outdoors are far too low to cause damage, but it can accumulate in enclosed spaces (the basements of houses, for example), where it can be inhaled and expose the lung cells to the isotope's alpha rays. People who are chronically exposed to radon, such as those who work in uranium mines, have an increased risk of lung cancer. As a result, the International Agency for Research on Cancer (IARC) has classified radon as a carcinogenic substance.

For the population in general, however, radon exposure is a much lower lung cancer risk factor than smoking, since the vast majority of people are exposed to doses of radon of 100 Bq/m³ or less. Just 0.5% of all deaths related to lung cancer are caused by radon alone, far behind the catastrophic impact of cigarettes, which cause 83% of deaths from this cancer (Figure 81). Smokers are also the people most likely to experience the damage caused by radon, with a mortality rate six times higher than that of nonsmokers. In other words, the harmful effect of radon on the risk of lung cancer could be reduced almost to zero simply by eliminating smoking.

Although radon is not a major cancer risk factor in non-smokers, people who want to know their level of exposure can consult the websites of their country's public health agencies to find out about the process to follow. Measuring radon levels is usually not expensive, and the corrective measures suggested in cases of above-normal exposure (aeration, ventilation and sealing) are usually sufficient to resolve the problem.

Putting Cancer to Sleep

Some people consider sleeping a "waste of time," an unproductive period when nothing happens, that must be limited to the bare minimum in order to get the most out of life. Denigrating

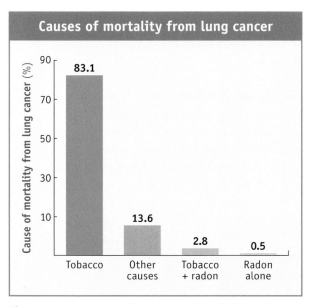

Figure 81

Adapted from Gray et al., 2009.

sleep is nothing new: for the ancient Greeks, sleeping was like a "little death" (Hypnos, the god of sleep, was the twin brother of Thanatos, the god of death), for "man, when asleep, is worth nothing," as Plato said.

This aversion to sleep is surprising; far from being a waste of time, sleep is essential for regenerating the body's energy reserves, eliminating metabolic waste from the brain produced by neuron activity to consolidate learning and memory, and enabling the immune system to function well. Many studies have also shown that sleep deficiency (fewer than 6 hours a night) increases the risk of premature death, as a result of an increase in several chronic diseases like heart disease, stroke or diabetes. These negative effects could in part be explained by the increased risk of obesity in people who get little sleep.

Studies done up to now in this field of research suggest that sleep disturbances are also associated with an increased risk for some cancers. For example, people who sleep fewer than 6 hours a night have an incidence of colorectal polyps, a major factor in colon cancer risk, 50% higher than those who sleep 7 hours. In elderly men who have trouble sleeping, the risk of prostate cancer increases significantly, especially for the most invasive forms of the disease. Similarly, menopausal women who suffer from insomnia are at higher risk of getting thyroid cancer, although this lack of sleep does not seem to influence their breast cancer risk.

The relationship between sleep and mortality risk is nonetheless complex. For example, people who work at night for long periods (20–30 years) have a roughly 50% higher risk of developing certain types of cancer (breast, prostate, colon, bladder and non-Hodgkin lymphoma) even when they get enough sleep. Several studies suggest that the change in the day/night cycle in these workers causes decreased melatonin secretion, melatonin being a hormone with several anticancer properties. These people must therefore pay special attention to adopting good lifestyle habits to make up as much as possible for the negative impact of upsetting their internal biological clock. Too much sleep (more than 9 hours) is also associated with

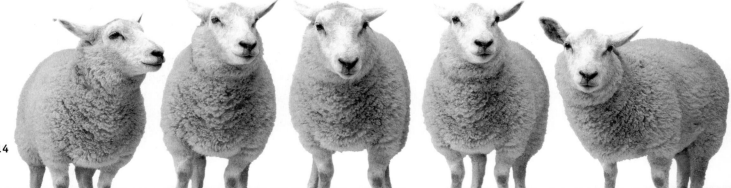

an increase in risk of chronic diseases and premature death. Colorectal cancer risk, for example, is greatly increased in people who sleep more than 9 hours a night, especially those who are overweight or snore. The longer period spent in bed by these people is likely a sign of poor quality sleep with frequent awakenings, which increases the secretion of cortisol, a stress hormone, and inflammatory molecules that can promote the growth of cancer cells. In addition, disturbed sleep is often the result of sleep-related respiratory problems called apneas, characterized by frequently interrupted breathing that causes fluctuations in blood pressure and creates inflammatory conditions. In addition to increasing the risk of cardiac events, apneas have recently been associated with increased cancer risk, possibly because they create favorable conditions for tumor vascularization, as well as for recruiting the inflammatory cells around them, creating a climate suitable for genetic mutations. Since excess body weight, and especially obesity, is the main cause of sleep apnea, these sleep disturbances likely contribute to the increase in cancer risk associated with being overweight.

We should spend a third of our lives sleeping: this is a rest period that is absolutely essential for preventing all chronic diseases, including cancer, and an indispensable ingredient for maintaining good health.

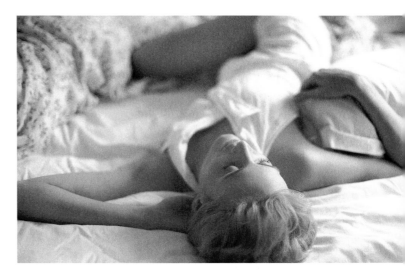

Psychological Factors

At the beginning of the Christian era, the physician Galen (ca. 129–201) maintained that melancholic women got cancer more often than those with a normal temperament. The influence of psychological factors on the onset of cancer is one of the most studied aspects of the disease, although no definitive link has been clearly established. For example, it has been suspected that certain character traits (extraversion, neurosis) might predispose some people to cancer because of the stress associated with the repression of negative emotions, but this kind of correlation has not been observed in large-scale studies. The impact of psychological trauma from painful life events has also been the subject of a great many studies, with some

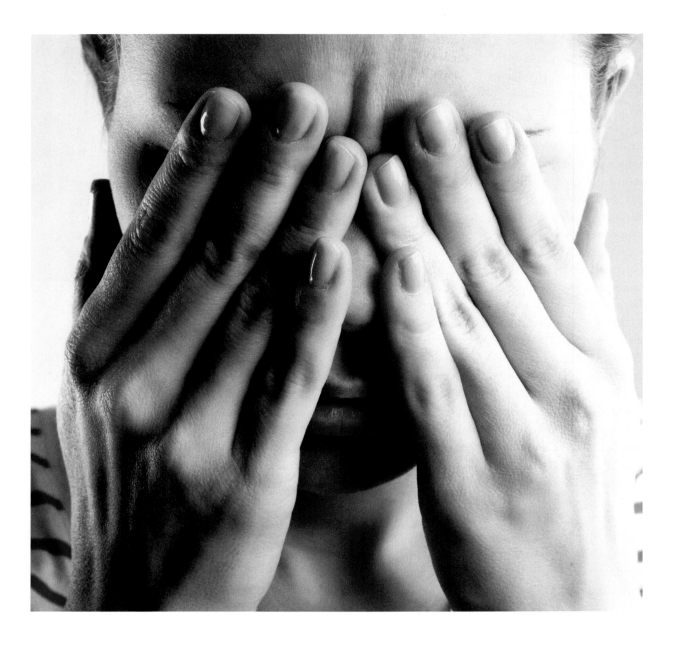

reporting an increased risk of breast cancer, for example, whereas in others this relationship was not observed. One of the most striking examples is the diagnosis of cancer in a child, one of the most intense sources of stress that can occur during a person's life. A study of 11,380 parents whose children have battled cancer indicates that these people show no increased cancer risk, and the mothers of these children do not seem to be at higher risk for breast cancer. Survivors of Nazi concentration camps, exposed to the worst ordeals a human being can be subjected to, have shown a life expectancy identical to, and in some cases superior to, that of people who did not experience this trauma. One recent study of 14,203 French participants indicates that there does not seem to be any relationship between the incidence of depressive episodes and the emergence of cancer, even in the case of severe depression, or between the stress of modern life and the incidence of several types of cancer, including breast cancer. Based on our current state of knowledge, the contribution of these psychological factors appears to be very slight, and much less pronounced than other aspects of our lifestyle. That said, stress is nonetheless recognized as a factor that speeds up the disappearance of telomeres, small regions at the ends of chromosomes that prevent our genetic material from being lost too quickly in the course of aging. Since more rapid telomere loss has been associated with the development

of several age-related diseases, the role of stress in the development of certain cancers cannot be totally excluded. From this perspective, there is no doubt that personality traits or tragic events can indirectly influence cancer risk if they are associated with unhealthy behaviors like smoking, alcohol abuse, physical inactivity or a bad diet.

It is also important to distinguish the impact of these psychological factors on the incidence of cancer from their impact on the disease's progression. It is well documented that most people who have survived cancer have difficulties sleeping well, with an insomnia rate three times higher than in the general population. Insomnia is considered more and more to be a major factor in the risk of depression, and several studies done in recent decades have shown that psychological suffering, whether in the form of anxiety, chronic depression or a lack of social support, is a factor associated with increased cancer risk. In people with cancer, therefore, psychological stress must be kept to a minimum, and better sleep is an essential step in this process. Studies have shown that changes in lifestyle, such as getting physical exercise or practicing activities like yoga, as well as psychological interventions like cognitive behavioral therapy, can in many cases improve the quality of sleep, and thus help people who are ill stay calmer in the face of this ordeal.

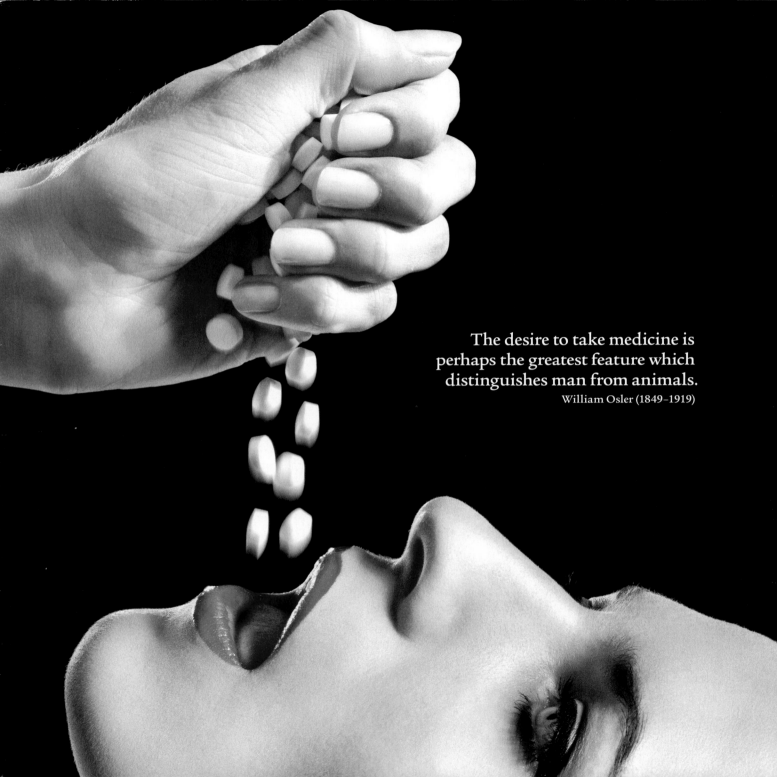

The desire to take medicine is perhaps the greatest feature which distinguishes man from animals.

William Osler (1849–1919)

Chapter 11

The Supplement Illusion

In recent decades, an extraordinary number of supplements have appeared on the market. Multivitamins, antioxidants, omega-3 supplements and plant extracts — all of these products are promoted as essential complements to the maintenance of good health, capable of making up for dietary imbalances. The supplement industry has long understood that the Western way of life is not conducive to the adoption of healthy lifestyle habits, whether because of the wide availability of poor quality foods, the lack of time available for preparing meals, or life circumstances that do not encourage physical activity. To remedy these limitations, an ever-growing number of so- called "natural" products have appeared, promising to solve the health problems caused by this lifestyle, without our having to reexamine our bad habits.

This "pillifying" of the diet is especially insidious when it claims to replace the beneficial effects of regularly eating fruits and vegetables. It has been known for several years that people who eat these plants regularly are in better health and have a lower risk of several types of cancer; this protection is due to phytoprotective compounds in plants that

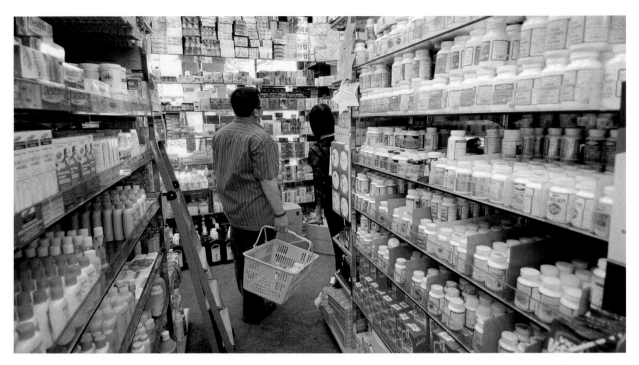

curb the progression of precancerous lesions. In the eyes of the industry, however, the positive impact of plants is mainly due to their vitamin and antioxidant content, so that a massive intake of some of these molecules, in the form of supplements, should also be good for health and produce anticancer effects that are exactly the same as, if not better than, those from plants. Yet this extrapolation has absolutely no scientific basis and can even prove dangerous, both because it creates a false sense of security and because it exposes people to quantities of certain substances that are far too high.

Too Much Is as Bad as Too Little

Preventing cancer by using vitamin and antioxidant supplements is a very attractive idea from a commercial point of view, but does not at all correspond to scientific reality. An impressive number of studies of large segments of the population have shown beyond any doubt that these supplements have no positive impact on health, whether it's a question of cancer, heart disease or life expectancy. The results of randomized trials are especially revealing in this regard, as these studies are considered to be the gold standard in clinical research (subjects are chosen at random, which minimizes statistical distortion). The conclusion drawn from the systematic analysis of several dozen of these studies is unequivocal: people who take supplements, whether multivitamins, vitamins C or E or beta-carotene, show no decrease in cancer risk.

Not only are these supplements ineffective in preventing cancer or other chronic diseases, but taking some of them is actually associated with an increase in mortality risk, according to several studies (Figure 82). Large amounts of vitamin E appear to be especially harmful, since they cause a marked increase in lung cancer risk among smokers when combined with beta-carotene, a sizable increase in prostate cancer risk, and a significant decrease in life expectancy. As the Renaissance physician Paracelsus wrote, "All things are poison, and nothing is without poison — only the dose determines what is not poison." In light of currently available data, supplements are perhaps one of the best modern illustrations of this truth.

Upsetting the Balance

The fact that antioxidant supplements have no protective effect, and that some of them are toxic, shows the danger of reducing a disease as complex as cancer to a simple battle between

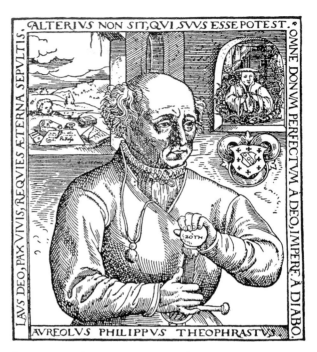

∧ Engraving of Paracelsus (1493–1541).

oxidants and antioxidants. Not all of the effects of free radicals on the body are harmful: regular physical exercise, for example, generates large quantities of free radicals, but it's still one of the main lifestyle factors involved in preventing the recurrence of several cancers. The generation of free radicals has also been associated with an increase in longevity in several organisms, a positive impact reversed by antioxidant supplements. The mechanisms responsible for these beneficial effects show the fundamental role played by free radicals when

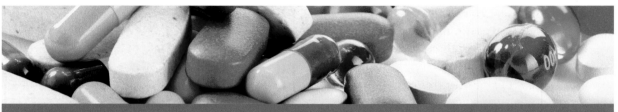

Examples of studies showing a negative impact from high doses of antioxidants		
Population	Antioxidants	Observed effects
29,133 smokers (50 and +)	**Vitamin E and beta-carotene**	↑ 16% in lung cancer risk ↑ 8% in risk of premature death
18,314 smokers and people exposed to asbestos	**Vitamin A and beta-carotene**	↑ 28% in lung cancer risk ↑ 17% in risk of premature death
Meta-analysis (20 studies, 211,818 people)	**Vitamins A, C and E, and beta-carotene**	↑ 16% in risk of mortality (beta-carotene + vitamin A) ↑ 6% in risk of mortality (beta-carotene + vitamin E)
Meta-analysis (19 studies, 135,967 people)	**Vitamin E**	↑ 4% in risk of premature death in excess of 400 UI/day
9,541 people (55 and +) at risk of heart disease	**Vitamin E**	↑ 13% in risk of heart failure
295,344 men (50-71)	**Multivitamins**	↑ 32% in prostate cancer risk with an excess of vitamins (more than seven times/week)
38,772 women (average age 62)	**Multivitamins and minerals**	↑ 2.4% in risk of premature mortality
35,533 men (50 and +)	**Vitamin E and selenium**	↑ 17% in risk of prostate cancer (vitamin E)
2,363 pregnant women at risk of preeclampsia	**Vitamins C and E**	↑ 2 times the risk of fetal loss or perinatal mortality

Figure 82

immune cells attack pathogens, as well as their participation in the process of eliminating abnormal precancerous cells through apoptosis.

Abnormally high concentrations of antioxidants taken in the form of supplements upset the delicate balance between the levels of free radicals normally generated by cells and the body's natural antioxidant defenses. As a result, instead of preventing cancer, these massive doses of antioxidants can paradoxically promote the development of the disease by interfering with the body's normal functioning, notably the systems involved in eliminating emerging tumors. In clinical practice, these supplements can also counteract the treatment of tumors with chemotherapy or radiotherapy, since it's the free radicals generated by these treatments that make it possible to shrink the tumor. Furthermore, the tumors that resist these treatments the most are often those with the highest antioxidant defense levels.

Some studies show that taking antioxidant supplements during and after radiotherapy treatment reduces the effectiveness of the radiation and significantly increases the risk of recurrence. Ultimately, antioxidant supplements are products of no use at all in preventing or treating cancer and can sometimes even be dangerous. Their use is therefore strongly discouraged.

The use of supplements implies that simple pills containing just one or a few molecules could replace a high-quality diet. This "medicalization" of the diet is very insidious, as it suggests that the act of eating only serves to supply the body with the vitamins and minerals it needs. So why worry about our diet if we can get these elements by swallowing a pill every morning? This is a ridiculous point of view, not only because it devalues the act of eating, but also because it's aiming at the wrong target: if there is one thing not missing from the modern diet, it's an adequate intake of vitamins and minerals! Our society does not suffer from a deficiency, but rather from dietary overabundance! And thanks to the fortification of dairy products and flours, even people who eat badly (junk food, processed products) usually have an adequate vitamin and mineral intake, which often even exceeds the daily recommended amounts. In this context, taking supplements to meet our

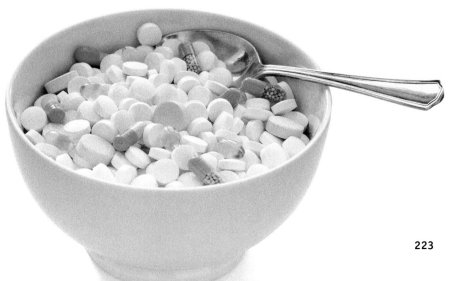

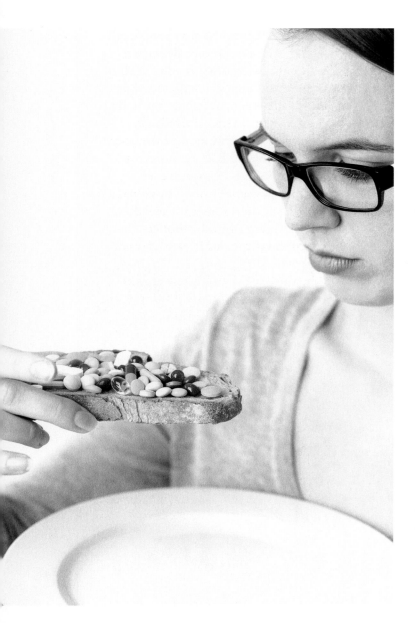

vitamin needs is a bit like adding a fifth foot to a chair: you may think it's more solid, but in reality its addition makes no difference whatsoever and adds nothing useful.

The false sense of security that can be attributed to taking supplements is dangerous, since the plants they are supposed to replace contain not only vitamins, but also, and most importantly, an impressive variety of phytochemical compounds that play a very important part in preventing chronic disease. For example, if a person decided not to eat any fruits or vegetables and to rely only on vitamin C supplements to meet his needs, he would supply his body with only this vitamin. Conversely, a person who avoids supplements and would rather bite into an apple will also get a substantial dose of vitamin C, but will at the same time absorb several dozen polyphenols naturally found in the skins of fruit (Figure 83). The biochemical diversity of plants is such that it's estimated that people who consume an abundance of fruits, vegetables, whole grains, nuts and certain beverages like green tea absorb 10,000 different phytochemical compounds every day, some of which perform well-documented anticancer activities. It goes without saying that no supplement will ever be able to reproduce this kind of biochemical diversity, nor make up for a plant-deficient diet.

Industrializing Health

If supplements are ineffective, how can we explain the fact that this industry is flourishing, with annual sales totaling $30 billion in the United States alone? This success depends first of all on the fact that most people (and even most health professionals) remain unaware of the negative results of these studies. Supplements must not be considered harmless substances, especially those delivering high doses of vitamin E. It's disturbing to realize that products containing 800 IU of vitamin E are on sale over the counter in drugstores, despite the fact that this quantity is twice as high as that associated with an increase in mortality in several studies.

A very wary approach must therefore be taken with regard to these products, especially when they lay claim to extraordinary benefits (see box p. 226). All of these supplements, of whatever kind, are made from only the tiniest portion of the active molecules in the foods they are taken from, and these cannot on their own reproduce the positive impact on

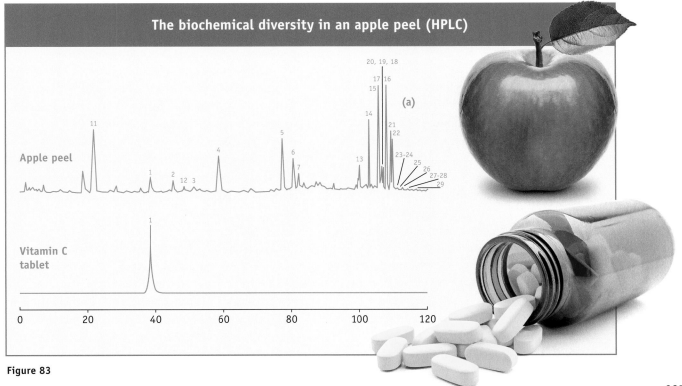

The biochemical diversity in an apple peel (HPLC)

Apple peel

Vitamin C tablet

Figure 83

False Claims

Avoid wasting time and money on ineffective supplements with no positive impact on health by being aware of these three never-fail signs.

Beware of extravagant health claims. When an effect seems too good to be true, that's because it isn't true! This is the case even when a celebrity is promoting it. Whether it's pills that make you lose 22 pounds (10 kg) in 1 week, miraculous "ionized" water or a new molecule that is supposed to protect the body from all diseases — all of these products are just modern versions of the snake oil sold by old-time charlatans.

Beware of exotic products. Just because a product is made from fruits or plants unfamiliar to us, or that come from faraway lands, does not mean it's blessed with miraculous properties. As the saying goes, "long ways, long lies..."

Beware of pseudoscientific jargon. To give credibility to a product, pseudoscientific terms are often used to describe it. But "laboratory tested," "100% natural," "native plant DNA," or other meaningless terms are first and foremost marketing tools developed by communications companies to attract a target audience.

health of the sum total of these molecules. A salmon is not just a long-chain omega-3 reservoir, and polyphenols are not just factors that make eating blueberries good for health. This reductionist approach, promoted by the industry, is destined to fail — all the more so because when these molecules are taken out of their natural context they are usually absorbed less efficiently by the intestine. In this regard, a recent study shows that the molecules in broccoli supplements are much less well absorbed than those in the actual vegetable; only the whole food can inhibit an enzyme that promotes cancer development. Even if they are absorbed, these molecules can nonetheless be damaged during the extraction or storage processes. Omega-3s, for example, are very fragile molecules, and studies have shown that supplements can contain a chemically modified form that is devoid of any activity and can even interfere with the action of omega-3s. Their pharmacological unavailability in tissues, the extracted molecules' biochemical instability, and the absence of product quality control are all reasons to banish these products from our daily lives.

It's therefore important to question the use of supplements and to realize that this is a dead-end strategy, from the standpoints both of health and of our relationship to food. In a way, taking supplements is the opposite of what diet has always represented in the evolution

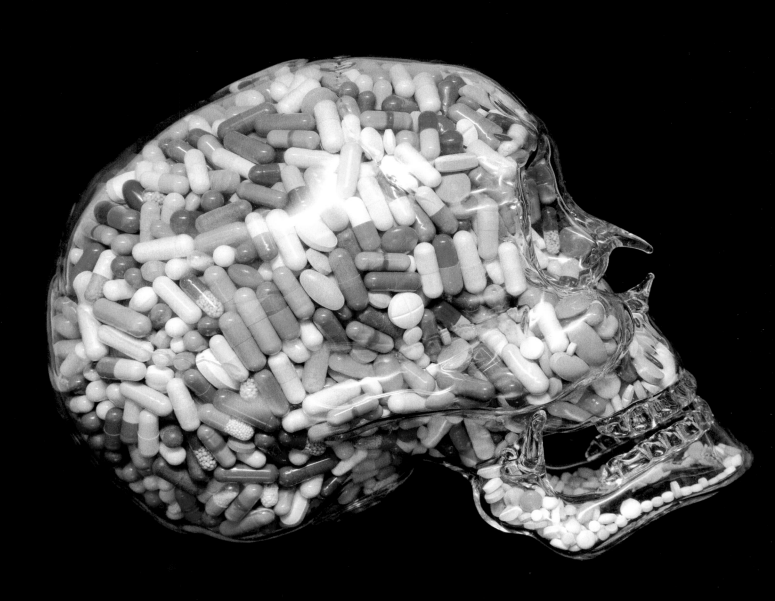

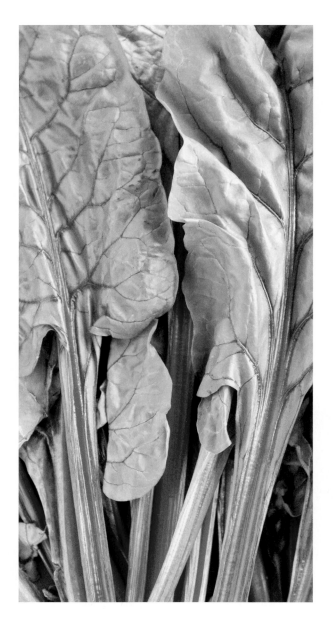

of the world's cultures: instead of trying to simplify what we eat, culinary traditions have on the contrary tended to become more complex, creating new flavors and textures by modifying daily foods. The fermenting of soy into miso, milk into yoghurt or cheese, or grapes into wine caused, in each case, major changes in the composition of the original foods, and these modifications are a source of benefits both for health and for gastronomic enjoyment.

Supplements can in no way replace the incredible biochemical diversity of the plant world; the interaction and synergy of the many molecules stemming from this biodiversity are the source of the protective effects of plants against cancer.

The Exception to the Rule

Although the use of supplements has to be called into question, we must nonetheless avoid being dogmatic and assuming that all supplements must be avoided without exception. For example, taking folic acid supplements around the time of conception is associated with a marked decrease in neural tube abnormalities (anencephalism and spina bifida), and these supplements are therefore strongly recommended to all women wanting to have a child.

In terms of cancer prevention, vitamin D is a supplement that can have protective effects, especially for inhabitants of the northern and southern latitudes. In contrast to other vitamins, which can be easily obtained from the diet, vitamin D is quite rare in nature and is mainly produced following exposure of the skin to the sun (see Chapter 9). Weak sunlight during the winter therefore means that many people have blood concentrations of vitamin D below recommended levels, which can lead to complex metabolic complications, given the important role of this vitamin in several physiological processes.

Since 1980, a number of studies have suggested that vitamin D deficiency might pave the way for the development of certain types of cancer. The first indicator of this came from observations showing that colon cancer mortality was higher in people who were least exposed to sunlight, such as residents of large cities or those in regions located at high latitudes. In the years since, no fewer than 15 types of cancer have been associated with lack of sun exposure, with this relationship being especially significant for colon, breast, prostate and non-Hodgkin lymphoma cancers. vitamin D seems to play the main role in this protective effect — a study has shown that postmenopausal women taking 1000 IU of vitamin D daily decreased their overall cancer risk by more than 60%,

and a decrease of 37% for lung cancer has also been observed after taking 400 IU a day. Similarly, people with a vitamin D deficiency (< 30 nmol/L) have a 42% higher risk of dying prematurely from cancer than those with normal levels of this vitamin.

Blood levels of vitamin D also seem to play an important role in the survival of people with cancer. Women with breast cancer whose vitamin D levels are too low (< 50 nmol/L) have almost twice the risk of recurrence following treatment and of dying from the disease. Similarly, people who receive a diagnosis of skin, prostate or colon cancer during the summer or fall, the time of year when vitamin D levels are highest, have a significantly greater likelihood of survival than those diagnosed in winter or spring. A similar impact is observed in patients with lung cancer: the survival rate without recurrence of an operation done in the summer on patients with high levels of vitamin D is twice that of the same treatment done in winter.

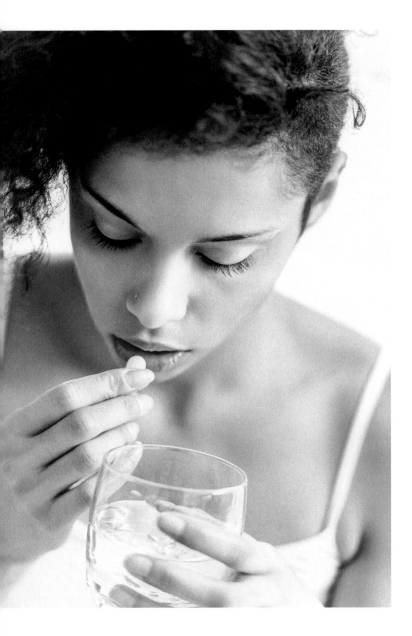

An Anticancer Vitamin

All of these observations strongly suggest that vitamin D deficiency increases the risk of getting certain kinds of cancer and that normalizing blood levels of this vitamin could be an inexpensive and safe way to reduce the incidence of cancer in the population and improve the likelihood of survival for people with the disease. Currently, most inhabitants of northern countries have an average vitamin D concentration of approximately 40 to 50 nmol/L, much lower than what is now considered to be the optimal level for this vitamin (75 nmol/L). The preventive potential of normalizing these levels is enormous: it's estimated that simply increasing vitamin D concentration by 25 nmol/L could reduce the incidence of all cancers by 17%, a level that could even be as high as 45% for cancers of the digestive system.

How to get there? An analysis of vitamin D levels in people who work outdoors in temperate regions shows concentrations of about 140 nmol/L, which corresponds to a daily intake of roughly 10,000 IU per day. In the summer, just 10 to 15 minutes of exposure is therefore enough for the skin to be able to synthesize sufficient vitamin D to reach recommended levels, without at the same time increasing the risk of skin cancer. The situation is very different from October to April, however, since weaker sunshine and colder temperatures greatly limit the skin's exposure to UV rays, especially in people who do not engage in winter sports. Milk is often considered a good way to make up for this lack of sunlight, but in reality the 100 or so IU of vitamin D in a glass of milk only raises blood levels of the vitamin by 2 or 3 nmol/L. Some foods, like salmon, tuna and shiitake mushrooms, are good sources of vitamin D (500–1000 IU per serving), but few people eat these foods regularly, and it would be false to think that they alone can make up for the winter deficiency in vitamin D. Because of all these factors, the use of supplements is really the only way to maintain adequate levels of vitamin D.

There are a wide variety of vitamin D supplements on the market, and this can make it hard to tell which are best for preventing cancer. First of all, make sure that the vitamin D is in the form of cholecalciferol (vitamin D_3), and not ergocalciferol (D_2); vitamin D_2 is a more unstable form from plants that is metabolized much less efficiently than vitamin D_3. Remember that toxic doses of this vitamin occur at 40,000 IU, far beyond our recommendations here. From a quantitative standpoint, even though a great many supplements on the market contain 400 IU of vitamin D_3, this dose would only lead to an increase of about 7 nmol/L. As a result, the Canadian Cancer Society, for example, recommends a daily fall and winter intake of 1000 IU.

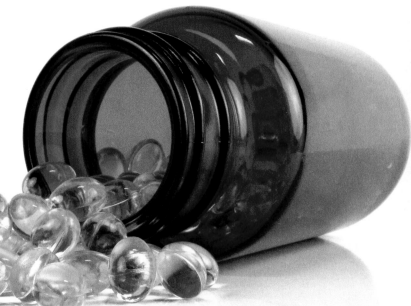

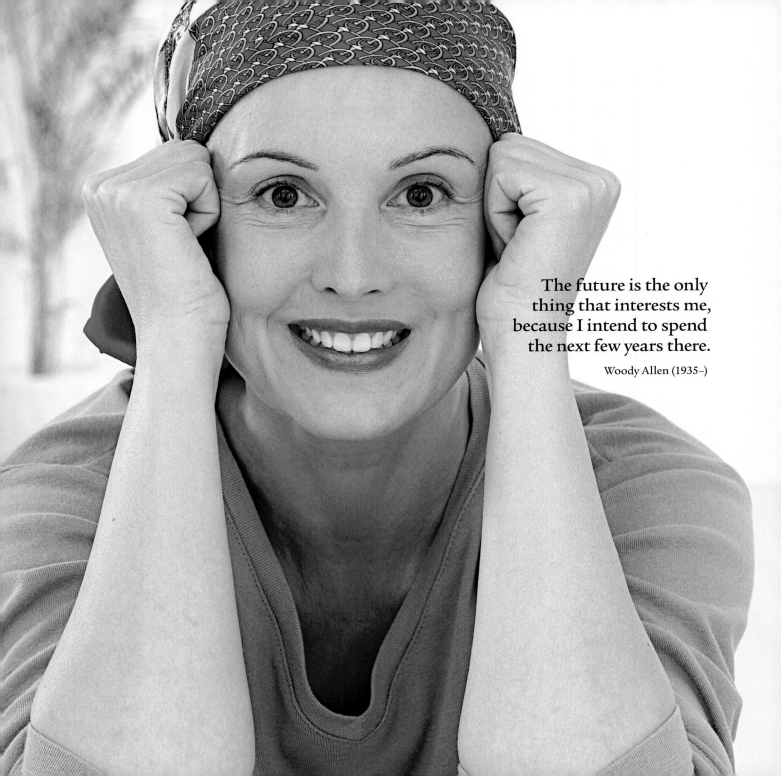

The future is the only
thing that interests me,
because I intend to spend
the next few years there.

Woody Allen (1935–)

Chapter 12

Surviving Cancer

Recommendation
Cancer survivors should follow the previously discussed recommendations for preventing the disease, to the letter.

Source: World Cancer Research Fund International

Medical advances in recent years have considerably changed the impact of cancer on society. Nowadays, the early detection of a number of cancers, combined with significant improvement in the effectiveness of treatments, means that two-thirds of people who have had cancer are still alive more than 5 years after diagnosis. With the aging of the population, it's estimated that the number of these cancer survivors will climb dramatically in the coming years, increasing from 25 million people in 2002 to nearly 70 million in 2050.

This improvement in survival rates is excellent news, but we must remain aware that the impact of cancer on people's lives does not stop when treatments do. In many, cancer leaves profound physical, psychological and emotional scars that can considerably impact their quality of life, one of the most significant of these being the fear of recurrence. This is a legitimate fear, as these people remain at high risk of getting the disease again during their lifetime. And cancers that reappear, sometimes several decades after the end of treatment, are even more dangerous than the initial cancers and are responsible for most deaths from the disease.

Indeed, one of the most frightening aspects of cancer is its unique ability to survive currently available treatments, whether these be very powerful cellular poisons, high

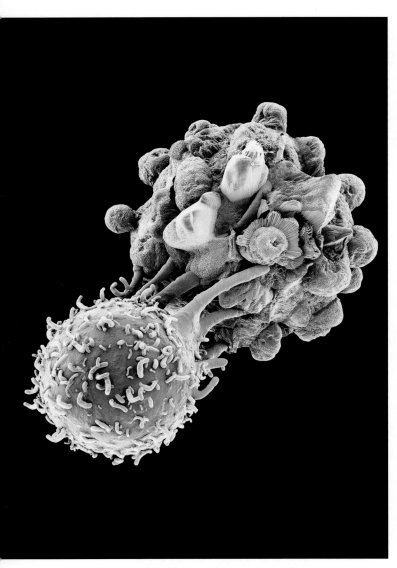

^ Illustration of a killer lymphocyte, on the left, attacking a cancer cell, on the right.

doses of radiation, or certain very specific drugs produced by human ingenuity and its unremitting efforts to treat the disease. Most of the time, these treatments succeed in eliminating almost all of the cancer cells, but the tiny number that manage to escape these attacks can remain incognito inside the body for several years, not unlike a hunted enemy that slowly regains its energy after a battle and plans its revenge. These dormant residual tumor cells are very dangerous, for in addition to having preserved the characteristics that enabled the initial tumor to invade a part of the body, these cells are now resistant to anticancer treatments and can thus prove invincible, as is usually the case when they recur. To survive cancer, the most important thing is therefore to prevent residual cells from reappearing, to do everything to make the body's internal environment as inhospitable as possible to them and prevent them from acquiring the characteristics necessary to express their destructive potential.

The good news is that this is a completely attainable goal. One of the most important discoveries in recent years has been to show that the lifestyle factors that prevent cancer from occurring in the first place, whether these be refraining from smoking, maintaining a healthy weight, eating a good diet or engaging in physical activity, can also play a predominant role in preventing recurrence (Figure 84).

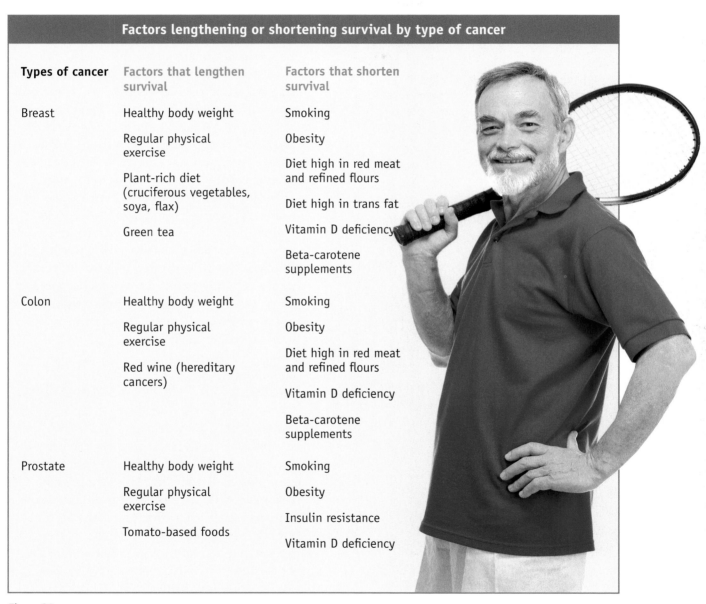

Factors lengthening or shortening survival by type of cancer

Types of cancer	Factors that lengthen survival	Factors that shorten survival
Breast	Healthy body weight	Smoking
	Regular physical exercise	Obesity
	Plant-rich diet (cruciferous vegetables, soya, flax)	Diet high in red meat and refined flours
	Green tea	Diet high in trans fat
		Vitamin D deficiency
		Beta-carotene supplements
Colon	Healthy body weight	Smoking
	Regular physical exercise	Obesity
	Red wine (hereditary cancers)	Diet high in red meat and refined flours
		Vitamin D deficiency
		Beta-carotene supplements
Prostate	Healthy body weight	Smoking
	Regular physical exercise	Obesity
	Tomato-based foods	Insulin resistance
		Vitamin D deficiency

Figure 84

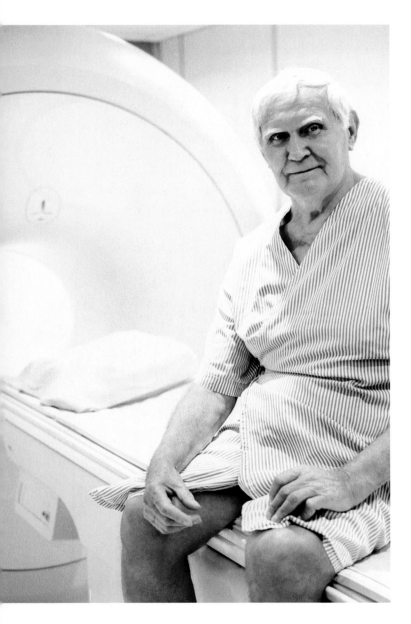

Thanks to the rigorous analysis done by the WCRF and the IARC, a list of lifestyle changes that can actually influence the risk of recurrence and increase life expectancy for people with cancer, especially breast, colon and prostate cancer, can be identified for the first time (Figure 84). The potential for preventing recurrence by applying these recommendations is still largely untapped, since very few cancer survivors change their lifestyles following diagnosis: fewer than 33% of them eat enough fruits and vegetables, and up to 70% for some cancers (breast, prostate) are overweight or obese. Just as for cancer prevention in general, simply putting the recommendations described in the preceding chapters into practice could therefore have extraordinary repercussions for survival after diagnosis and treatment for several types of cancer.

Smoking: It's Never Too Late to Quit

Some studies indicate that barely half of patients who receive a diagnosis of cancer quit smoking, even when the disease is a direct consequence of smoking. This attitude of course reflects nicotine's strong addictive power, but also a kind of resignation on the part of smokers in the face of their condition, almost as though quitting smoking would be a futile effort, since the damage caused by tobacco is already done and is irreversible. The reality is very different, since the risk of dying is 76% higher for people who keep on smoking after a cancer diagnosis than for those who stop. The negative impact of tobacco is not limited to lung cancer, with the risk of mortality for smokers also being higher for cancer of the prostate, colon and vulva, as well as for leukemia and malignant melanoma. Recent studies also indicate that women who continue to smoke after a diagnosis of breast cancer have a risk of dying prematurely three times higher than those who quit.

Although essential for decreasing the incidence of cancer, quitting smoking is also a key step in improving the survival chances of people who already have it.

A Weight-Loss Diet for Cancer Cells

Obesity is a cancer risk factor, but several studies also indicate that being overweight reduces the life expectancy of people who have already had certain types of cancer. For example, obese women with breast cancer have a 33% greater risk of recurrence than thin women. This phenomenon is even more pronounced in younger women, with obesity at age 20 being associated with more than twice the mortality risk. Being obese at the time of diagnosis is also associated with a lower survival rate for people with colon or prostate cancer. In the

case of the latter, men who are overweight (with a BMI between 25 and 29) already have a 50% higher risk of dying from their cancer than men who are thin (with a BMI below 25), and this increased risk is as high as 170% in obese men (Figure 85). The negative impact of excess body weight on the chance of survival is all the more serious if accompanied by high insulin levels, common in people who are overweight or obese; people with a BMI over 25 and a high level of insulin are four times as likely to die from this cancer.

In addition to playing a major role in the incidence of

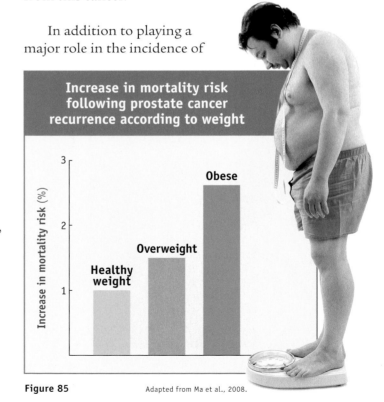

Increase in mortality risk following prostate cancer recurrence according to weight

Increase in mortality risk (%)

Obese

Overweight

Healthy weight

Figure 85   Adapted from Ma et al., 2008.

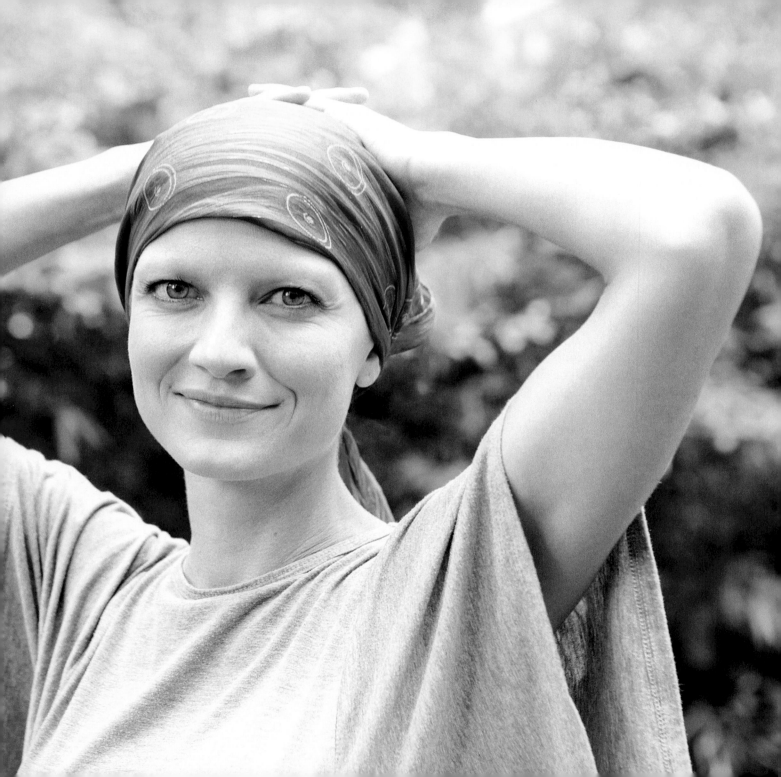

excess weight and obesity, eating too many processed foods high in fat and sugar could, in and of itself, encourage some cancers to recur. For example, women who eat the largest amounts of foods high in saturated fats and trans fat after a diagnosis of invasive breast cancer are up to 78% more likely to die prematurely, and consuming foods with a high glycemic index, containing for example added simple sugars, is associated with twice the risk of recurrence and mortality in patients with stage III colorectal cancer. As for prostate cancer, these recurrences are likely a direct consequence of the increase in insulin associated with this kind of diet, which encourages the growth of residual cancer cells.

Consuming overprocessed industrial foods high in sugar and fat thus promotes obesity and the development of cancer, both in the population as a whole and in people with the disease, and maintaining normal body weight should be a goal for everyone who wants to reduce the risk of recurrence and improve their life expectancy.

Red Meat

In addition to increasing the risk of colorectal cancer, eating red meat and processed meats is also associated with a significant decrease in survival in patients with this disease. People who regularly eat these foods after diagnosis have almost twice the risk of dying from this cancer. And these harmful effects can be magnified by the fact that red meat and processed meat are often part of a "Western-type" diet, high in sugar and refined flours. Studies indicate that these kinds of food habits triple the risk of mortality in people with colorectal or breast cancer, compared with people who adopt a healthier diet, low in red meat but high in plants.

Plant Chemotherapy

As the Arab proverb says so well, "too much of something is a lack of something." Thus, a high intake of industrial foods and meat almost always accompanies a plant-food deficiency. Cancer survivors are no exception to this rule, since most only slightly increase their plant-food consumption after diagnosis. Some studies even indicate that up to 90% of them have an intake of fruits, vegetables and whole grains below the minimum of five recommended servings.

This deficiency is concerning, as several research studies suggest that the anticancer molecules in plants slow down the development of the microscopic tumors that form spontaneously during our lifetimes, and indicate that these molecules might even do the same for the dormant microtumors in cancer survivors. In this vein, it's quite remarkable that several foods known to decrease the incidence of certain cancers have a similar positive impact on recurrence and mortality risks. For example, a study of 9,574 women with invasive breast cancer indicated that in those who regularly ate foods based on soy, an isoflavone source known to decrease cancer risk, the risk of recurrence decreased by about 30%, and this in no way interfered with the effectiveness of tamoxifen or anastrozole. Initial fears about soy increasing the risk of recurrence are thus completely unfounded; phytoestrogens can, on the contrary, prove to be valuable allies in improving the prognosis for breast cancer. Very encouraging protective effects have also been observed with respect to lignans, another class of phytoestrogens found in large amounts in flaxseed and whole grains, with a 70% reduction in mortality in menopausal women who had had breast cancer.

The cruciferous vegetables are another class of plants that could significantly improve the prognosis for some cancers. For example, the isothiocyanates formed after eating these vegetables are powerful bladder cancer inhibitors owing to their presence in large quantities in the urine. Recent observations indicate that people with this cancer who eat just one serving of broccoli a week see their risk of dying from this cancer decrease by 60%. Similar protection has been seen in breast cancer survivors, with people who eat three servings of cruciferous vegetables a week having half the recurrence rate.

The dramatic decrease in recurrence caused by phytoestrogens and cruciferous vegetables underlines the importance of modifying our food habits to give these exceptional foods a prominent place. A better prognosis has also been observed in prostate cancer patients who consume tomato-based products, as well as in women who have fought breast cancer and who drink green tea (more than 3 cups a day), and other protective plants will likely be identified in the coming years. For people who have survived cancer, an increased intake of plant-based foods is thus essential for preventing recurrence, a kind of nontoxic chemotherapy in which the anticancer molecules of several plants interact with residual microtumors and keep them in a latent and harmless state.

A Whirlwind of Cancer-Fighting Activities!

Human physiology is designed for movement, so it's not surprising that physical activity offers many health benefits, from the physical (aerobic capacity, strength, flexibility), metabolic (glycemia control) and mental (stress reduction, cognitive functions) points of view. These benefits are especially important for people who have had cancer, since better physical and psychological endurance can prove indispensable in dealing with the many difficulties linked to the diagnosis and treatment of the disease. Several organizations, including the American Cancer Society, the World Cancer Research Fund and the American College of Sports Medicine, recommend

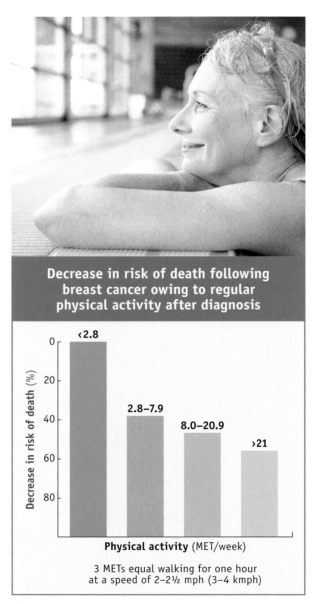

Decrease in risk of death following breast cancer owing to regular physical activity after diagnosis

3 METs equal walking for one hour at a speed of 2–2½ mph (3–4 kmph)

Figure 86 Adapted from Holick et al., 2008.

that people with cancer perform at least 10 metabolic equivalents (10 METs) a week, which corresponds to 2½ hours of moderate-intensity physical activity, like fast walking, to reduce mortality risk.

These recommendations are based on a large number of studies that conclude unequivocally that cancer survivors who are the most physically active are also those who live the longest. This protective effect is especially well documented for breast cancer, with women who are active (a minimum of 9 METs a week) having their overall mortality reduced by half, compared with those who are inactive (Figure 86). Moderate physical activity is enough to cause a significant increase in survival, but studies suggest that these benefits are even more pronounced in the most active people (> 20 METs per week). Even though the prognosis is even better for women who were already active before receiving a diagnosis of breast cancer, it's nonetheless never too late to get moving. People who were inactive before getting sick, but who decide to incorporate regular physical activity into their habits following diagnosis, have a 45% lower risk of dying prematurely than if they stayed inactive. Conversely, people who were physically active but who decreased their activity level following diagnosis see their risk of mortality increase by 400%. Similar results have been observed

in colon cancer survivors, with mortality decreased by half in those most active after diagnosis, in both men and women, although a higher activity level (> 20 METs per week) seems to be necessary to generate protective effects. An increase in survival rates owing to physical activity in people who have had prostate, ovarian (in nonobese women) and brain cancer has also been observed, but this still has to be better characterized.

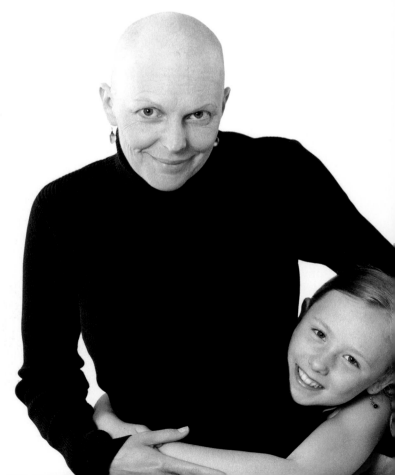

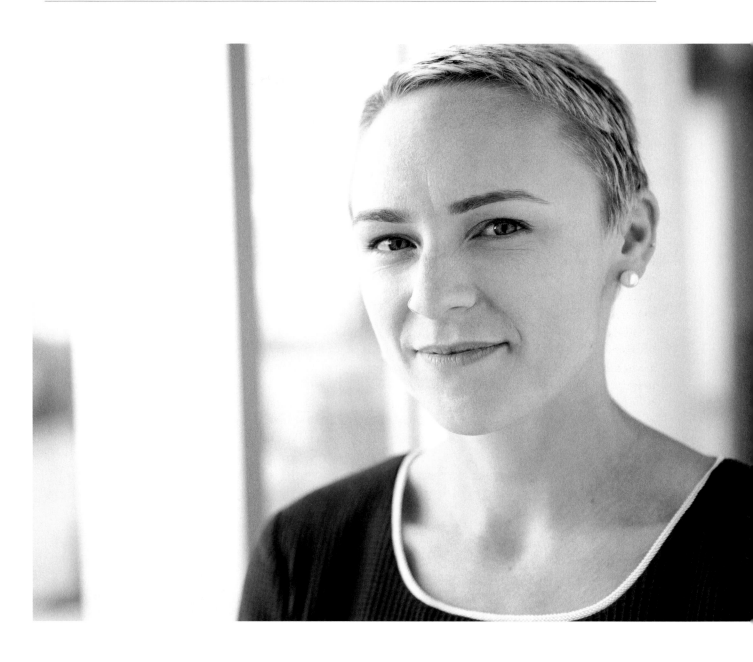

The positive impact of physical activity on survival reflects the many metabolic and hormonal effects associated with body movement. For example, exercise is the best protective agent for diabetes, and the prevention of this disease definitely plays a role, given the sharp rise in mortality in cancer survivors who are diabetic. Physical activity also improves immune function and regulates the levels of several hormones and inflammatory molecules involved in cancer development (insulin, estrogens, adiponectin, IL-6), two aspects that might contribute to its beneficial effects. However, whatever the mechanisms at play, no other discovery in recent years has as much potential as physical activity for improving both quality of life and life expectancy in people who have had cancer. Remember that being physically active does not mean it is absolutely necessary to perform feats of athleticism or become a fitness fanatic. In every study showing an increase in survival, fast walking, available to everyone, was the most commonly adopted activity. Physical activity of whatever kind should be considered an essential component of cancer survivors' daily routines.

To Drink or Not to Drink?

Few substances have such complex effects on health as alcohol, whose well-documented benefits for cardiovascular health are counterbalanced by a parallel increase in risk of certain cancers, especially breast cancer. This is a particularly problematic situation for women with this cancer who were in the habit of drinking moderately before the diagnosis: is the risk of recurrence associated with alcohol greater than its positive effects on the decrease in mortality linked to heart disease?

Studies done up to now are fairly reassuring and indicate that women who consume alcohol moderately after a diagnosis of breast cancer show no increased risk of mortality. Some studies have even reported a positive impact associated with moderate alcohol consumption (one glass a day), with a decrease in mortality, compared with women who don't drink. As is the case for the population in general, currently available data thus indicate that the impact of alcohol on mortality risk appears to be the same in women with breast cancer as in the general population; in other words, moderate alcohol consumption slightly increases the risk of dying from cancer but reduces to a greater degree the mortality risk linked to heart disease, the main cause of death in menopausal women. For all women, whether or not they have had breast cancer, drinking alcohol is therefore a very personal decision that depends on each person's comfort zone. For those who choose to drink, red wine seems to be the best choice, as its impact on several types of cancer, especially colon cancer, is less negative and sometimes even beneficial (see p. 158). It's interesting to note, for example, that drinking red wine has been associated with longer survival in patients with hereditary colorectal cancer.

Foods Instead of Supplements

Supplements are especially popular among cancer patients, who are usually more inclined to try different combinations of supplements to fight the disease. As many as 80% take one supplement or another, a habit that is particularly common among women and more educated people. Multivitamins, calcium, vitamin D and antioxidants are the most popular.

The popularity of supplements in no way reflects their clinical usefulness. The great many studies that have examined the effect of various supplements indicate that these products do not improve the prognosis or overall survival of patients, and might even in some cases increase mortality risk. For example, the use of antioxidant or vitamin A supplements is not associated with a decrease in mortality in cancer patients, nor does taking a wide array of supplements or multivitamins improve the survival of people with breast or colon cancer.

Furthermore, several studies suggest that carotenoid supplements could have major negative side effects for cancer survivors. A recent study showed that women who took these supplements following a diagnosis of breast cancer had twice as high a risk of mortality, an observation that corroborates the results of earlier studies indicating that beta-carotene increased colorectal adenoma recurrence in smokers and people who drink alcohol. Similarly, patients receiving radiation for the treatment of head and neck cancer who take high doses of vitamin E (400 IU a day) considerably increase their mortality risk.

All of these observations illustrate the degree to which people with cancer can, in many cases, considerably improve their likelihood of surviving the disease. One of the best examples is breast cancer, where a large number of studies have clearly shown that simple daily actions, like regular physical activity, maintaining a healthy body weight, and adopting a diet rich in plants, especially those high in anticancer molecules, can significantly reduce the risk of recurrence and death (Figure 87).

Examples of studies showing the importance of lifestyle for breast cancer survivors

Lifestyle parameter measured	Number of participants	Impact on survival	Reference
Factors that improve survival			
Physical activity	4,482	↓ 50% deaths all causes ↓ 50% deaths from breast cancer	Holick et al., 2008.
Consumption of fruits, vegetables and whole grains	1,901 2,522	↓ 65% deaths all causes ↓ 25% deaths all causes ↓ 30% recurrences of breast cancer	Kwan et al., 2009. Vrieling et al., 2013.
Consumption of soy	11,206	↓ 15% deaths all causes ↓ 25% recurrences of breast	Chi et al. 2013.
Consumption of foods high in lignans	1,122	↓ 50% deaths all causes ↓ 75% deaths from breast cancer	McCann et al., 2010.
Consumption of cruciferous vegetables	3,080	↓ 50% recurrences of breast cancer (women treated with tamoxifen)	Thomson et al., 2011.
Consumption of green tea	5,617	↓ 25% recurrences of breast cancer	Ogunleye et al., 2010.
Factors that decrease survival			
Being overweight	1,254	↑ 50% deaths all causes for BMI >30	Abrahamson et al., 2006.
"Western" diet (red meat, processed meats and refined flours)	1,901 2,522	↑ 200% deaths all causes ↑ 360% deaths all causes	Kwan et al., 2009. Vrieling et al., 2013.
Diet high in trans fat **Diet high in saturated fat**	4,441 4,441	↑ 78% deaths all causes ↑ 74% deaths all causes	Beasley et al., 2011.
Smoking	2,265	↑ 100% deaths related to breast cancer ↑ 400% deaths all causes	Braithwaite et al., 2012.
Vitamin D deficiency	512	↑ 94% recurrences of breast cancer ↑ 73% deaths related to breast cancer (vitamin D < 50 nmol/L on diagnosis)	Goodwin et al., 2009.

Figure 87

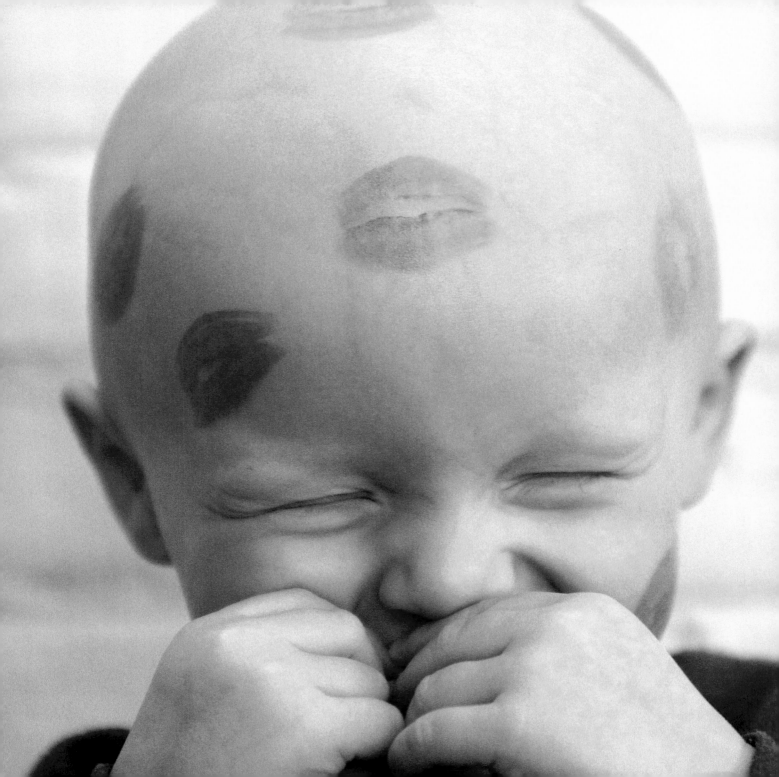

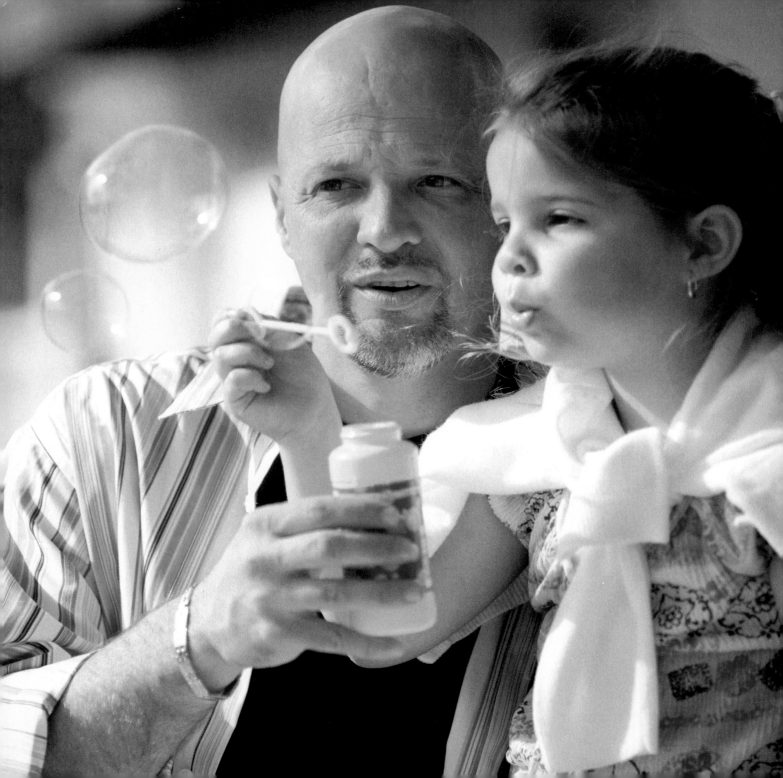

Conclusion

Cancer is now the leading cause of death in several Western societies, where it is estimated that in the near future 50% of the population will be at risk of experiencing this scourge. Lifestyle has an extraordinary impact on the likelihood of preventing or surviving the disease, and a number of very simple daily behaviors can contribute in remarkable ways to preventive efforts. We must not wait passively to be diagnosed before reevaluating our lifestyle and choosing behaviors that lead to healthier habits.

Even without having a clinically confirmed cancer, everyone has many precancerous lesions that form spontaneously in the body throughout life. In the vast majority of cases, lifestyle is what determines whether these lesions remain in a microscopic state, slow growing and harmless, or whether, on the contrary, they will evolve into mature tumors. Although the human body has an innate resistance to cancer, thanks to natural mechanisms that create inhospitable conditions for these lesions and hinder their development, these defense mechanisms must nonetheless be allowed to function optimally, so that tumors remain latent and benign.

We are not therefore as helpless in the face of cancer as we might think, and daily behaviors that have an enormous influence on the statistical risk of getting this disease can be adopted. The potential for prevention is quite remarkable. It is estimated that the majority of deaths from cancer could be avoided by applying the recommendations of the major agencies in the fight against cancer, as explained in this book.

Cancer survivors, for their part, can also take their fate into their own hands after therapeutic intervention, and undertake concrete action to improve their chances of survival in the long term. Adopting a lifestyle inspired by recent population studies, a change within everyone's reach, can play a leading role in this endeavor.

Preventing cancer and its recurrence by changing lifestyle habits is truly a revolution in our approach to cancer. In the past, our reflex was often to rely solely on medical intervention, hoping that the discovery of more effective treatments would finally make it possible to win the battle. The enormous individual and societal burden still imposed by cancer indicates that this approach has its limits and that by itself it cannot meet our expectations.

Preventing cancer is a realistic and concrete concept. In our current state of knowledge, adopting a preventive attitude is a very important complementary approach for making significant progress in the battle against this terrifying enemy, helping us reduce the likelihood of getting cancer while increasing our chances of surviving it with the best possible quality of life.

Chapter 1

Vogelstein, B. et al. "Cancer genome landscapes," *Science* 2013; 339: 1546-58.

Siegel, R. et al. "Cancer statistics, 2014," *CA Cancer J Clin* 2014; 64: 9-29.

Van Panhuis, W.G. et al. "Contagious diseases in the United States from 1888 to the present," *N Engl J Med* 2013; 369: 2152-2158.

Ford, E.S. et al. "Explaining the decrease in U.S. deaths from coronary disease, 1980-2000," *N Engl J Med* 2007; 356: 2388-98.

Greaves, M. "Darwinian medicine: a case for cancer," *Nature Rev Cancer* 2007; 7: 213-221.

www.cancer.ca/en/cancer-information/cancer-101/cancer-statistics-at-a-glance/?region=bc#ixzz2jh6lDa3X

Frank, S.A. "Evolution in health and medicine Sackler colloquium: Somatic evolutionary genomics: mutations during development cause highly variable genetic mosaicism with risk of cancer and neurodegeneration," *Proc Natl Acad Sci USA* 2010; 107: 1725-1730.

Li, R. et al. "Somatic point mutations occurring early in development: a monozygotic twin study," *J Med Genet* 2014 Jan; 51(1): 28-34; doi: 10.1136/jmedgenet-2013-101712.

www.cancer.ca/en/cancer-information/cancer-type/pancreatic/statistics/?region=bc

DeGregori, J. "Challenging the axiom: does the occurrence of oncogenic mutations truly limit cancer development with age?," *Oncogene* 2013; 32: 1869-75.

Nielsen, M. et al. "Breast cancer and atypia among young and middle-aged women: a study of 110 medicolegal autopsies," *Br J Cancer* 1987; 56: 814-9.

Sakr, W.A. et al. "The frequency of carcinoma and intraepithelial neoplasia of the prostate in young male patients," *J Urol* 1993; 150: 379-385.

Renehan, A.G. et al. "The prevalence and characteristics of colorectal neoplasia in acromegaly," *J Clin Endocrinol Metab* 2000; 85: 3417-3424.

Jonason, A.S. et al. "Frequent clones of p53-mutated keratinocytes in normal human skin," *Proc Natl Acad Sci USA* 1996; 93: 14025-14029.

Manser, R.L. et al. "Incidental lung cancers identified at coronial autopsy: implications for overdiagnosis of lung cancer by screening," *Respir Med* 2005; 99: 501-507.

Cubilla, A.L. and P.J. Fitzgerald. "Morphological lesions associated with human primary invasive nonendocrine pancreas cancer," *Cancer Res* 1976; 36: 2690-8.

Harach, H.R. et al. "Occult papillary carcinoma of the thyroid: a 'normal' finding in Finland. A systematic autopsy study," *Cancer* 1985; 56: 531-538.

Greaves, M.F. et J.Wiemels. "Origins of chromosome translocations in childhood leukemia," *Nat Rev Cancer* 2003; 3: 1-10.

Bose, S. et al. "The presence of typical and atypical BCR-ABL fusion genes in leukocytes of normal individuals: biologic significance and implications for the assessment of minimal residual disease," *Blood* 1998; 92: 3362-3367.

Brown, L.M. et al. "Incidence of adenocarcinoma of the esophagus among white Americans by sex, stage, and age," *J Natl Cancer Inst* 2008; 100: 1184-7.

Sørensen, T.I. et al. "Genetic and environmental influences on premature death in adult adoptees," *N Engl J Med* 1988; 318: 727-732.

http://massgenomics.org/2011/05/inflammation-genetic-instability-and-cancer.html

Nelson, N.J. "Migrant studies aid the search for factors linked to breast cancer risk," *J Natl Cancer Inst* 2006; 98: 436-8.

Shin, H.R. et al. "Recent trends and patterns in breast cancer incidence among Eastern and Southeastern Asian women," *Cancer Causes Control* 2010; 21: 1777-85.

Jung, Y.S. et al. "Nation-wide Korean breast cancer data from 2008 using the Breast Cancer Registration Program," *J Breast Cancer* 2011; 14: 229-236.

King, M.C. et al. "Breast and ovarian cancer risks due to inherited mutations in BRCA1 and BRCA2," *Science* 2003; 302: 643-6.

Nkondjock, A. et al. "Diet, lifestyle and BRCA-related breast cancer risk among French-Canadians," *Breast Cancer Res Treat* 2006; 98: 285-294.

Tryggvadottir, L. et al. "Population-based study of changing breast cancer risk in Icelandic BRCA2 mutation carriers, 1920-2000," *J Natl Cancer Inst* 2006; 98: 116-122.

Loeb, L.A. "Mutator phenotype may be required for multistage carcinogenesis," *Cancer Res* 1991; 51: 3075-3079.

Almog, N. "Genes and regulatory pathways involved in persistence of dormant micro-tumors," *Adv Exp Med Biol* 2013; 734: 3-17.

Tian, X. et al. "High-molecular-mass hyaluronan mediates the cancer resistance of the naked mole rat," *Nature* 2013; 499: 346-9.

Sjöblom, T. et al. "The consensus coding sequences of human breast and colorectal cancers," *Science* 2006; 314: 268-274.

Yatani, R. et al. "Latent prostatic carcinoma: Pathological and epidemiological aspects," *Jpn J Clin Oncol* 1989; 19: 319-326.

Watanabe, M. et al. "Comparative studies of prostate cancer in Japan versus the United States. A review," *Urol Oncol* 2000; 5: 274-283.

Center, M.M. et al. "International variation in prostate cancer incidence and mortality rates," *Eur Urol* 2012; 61: 1079-92.

http://globocan.iarc.fr/factsheets/cancers/colorectal.asp

Welch, H.G. and W.C. Black. "Overdiagnosis in cancer.," *J Natl Cancer Inst* 2010; 102: 605-613.

http://science.education.nih.gov/supplements/nih1/cancer/guide/understanding3.htm

Colditz, G.A. et al. "Applying what we know to accelerate cancer prevention," *Sci Transl Med* 2012; 4: 127rv4.

Fineberg, H.V. "The paradox of disease prevention: celebrated in principle, resisted in practice," *JAMA* 2013; 310: 85-90.

Inoue-Choi, M. et al. "Adherence to the WCRF/AICR guidelines for cancer prevention is associated with lower mortality among older female cancer survivors," *Cancer Epidemiol Biomarkers Prev* 2013; 22: 792-802.

Arab, L. et al. "Adherence to World Cancer Research Fund/American Institute for Cancer Research lifestyle recommendations reduces prostate cancer aggressiveness among African and Caucasian Americans," *Nutr Cancer* 2013; 65: 633-43.

Vergnaud, A.C. et al. "Adherence to the World Cancer Research Fund/American Institute for Cancer Research guidelines and risk of death in Europe: results from the European Prospective Investigation into Nutrition and Cancer cohort study," *Am J Clin Nutr* 2013; 97: 1107-20.

Hastert, T.A. et al. "Adherence to WCRF/AICR cancer prevention recommendations and risk of postmenopausal breast cancer," *Cancer Epidemiol Biomarkers Prev* 2013; 22: 1498-508.

Chapter 2

Benedict, C. *Golden-Silk Smoke: A History of Tobacco in China, 1550-2010*, University of California Press, 352 pages, 2011.

Winter, J.C. *Tobacco Use by Native North Americans: Sacred Smoke and Silent Killer*, University of Oklahoma Press, 454 pages, 2000.

www.larecherche.fr/idees/back-to-basic/tabac-01-05-2009-87948

Ferland, C. "Mémoires tabagiques. L'usage du tabac, du xve siècle à nos jours," *Drogues, santé et société* 2007; 6: 17-48.

Ferland, C. "Une pratique "sauvage"? Le tabagisme de l'Ancienne à la Nouvelle-France, xviie-xviiie siècles," in *Tabac et Fumées. Regards multidisciplinaires et indisciplinés sur le tabagisme, xve-xxe siècles*, Presses de l'Université Laval, 236 pages, 2007.

King James I of England. *A Counter-Blaste to Tobacco*, 1604.

Surowiecki, J. "Up in Smoke," *The New Yorker*, 21 novembre 2005.

Rival, N. *Tabac, miroir du temps*, Perrin, 281 pages, 1981.

www.cigares.com/blog/histoire-cigare/

www.les-derniers-romanov.com/histoire.php

Osipova, A. "Smoke of the Motherland," *Russian Life*, January–February 2007.

Blakeslee, S. "Nicotine: harder to kick... than heroin," *The New York Times*, 29 mars 1987.

http://bdc.aege.fr/public/Analyse_pratiques_Guerre_information_industrie_tabac.pdf

Pampel, F.C. *Tobacco Industry and Smoking. Facts on file*, 314 pages, 2009.

Cigarette Consumption, United States, 1900-2007. *Tobacco Outlook Report*, Economic Research Service, U.S. Dept. of Agriculture.

www.tobaccoatlas.org

Nielsen, S.S. et al. "Nicotine from edible Solanaceae and risk of Parkinson disease," *Ann Neurol* 2013 (9 mai); doi: 10.1002/ana.23884.

Henningfield, J.E. "More on the nicotine content of vegetables," *N Engl J Med* 1993; 329: 1581-82.

www.tis-gdv.de/tis_e/ware/genuss/tabak/tabak.htm

Siegmund, B. et al. "Determination of the nicotine content of various edible nightshades (Solanaceae) and their products and estimation of the associated dietary nicotine intake," *J Agric Food Chem* 1999; 47: 3113-3120.

Domino, E.F. et al. "The nicotine content of common vegetables," *N Engl J Med* 1993; 329: 437.

Wigand, J.S. *Additives, cigarette design and tobacco product regulation: a report to World Health Organization*, 2006 (www.jeffreywigand.com/WHOFinal.pdf)

Vey, T. "Des enfants produisent du tabac pour Philip Morris," *Le Figaro*, 16 juillet 2010.

Gilbert, S.G. *A Small Dose of Toxicology: The Health Effects of Common Chemicals*, CRC Press, 280 pages, 2004.

Tassin, J.P. et al. "Un nouveau concept explicatif de la pharmaco-dépendance: le découplage des neurones sérotoninergiques et noradrénergiques," http://dx.doi.org/10.1051/medsci/20062210798

http://lecerveau.mcgill.ca/flash/i/i_03/i_03_cr/i_03_cr_par/i_03_cr_par.html

Xiu, X. et al. "Nicotine binding to brain receptors requires a strong cation-pi interaction," *Nature* 2009; 458: 534-7.

http://sante.lefigaro.fr/dossier/tabac/comment-arreter/boite-outils-pour-arreter-fumer

Fowler, J.S. et al. "Inhibition of monoamine oxidase B in the brains of smokers," *Nature* 1996; 379: 733-736.

Tassin, J.P. "Dépendance au tabac: pour en finir avec la nicotine," *Slate*, 25 mars 2013.

Budney, A.J. et al. "Marijuana dependence and its treatment," *Addict Sci Clin Pract* 2007; 4: 4-16.

Mathias, R.G. "Comment aborder l'usage des drogues au Canada: une nouvelle perspective sur l'usage des drogues par les Canadiens," www.parl.gc.ca/content/sen/committee/371/ille/presentation/mathias-f.htm

www.sante.public.lu/fr/maladies-traitements/010-maladies/tete/maladies-tete/dependance-a-nicotine/index.html

Hecht, S.S. "Tobacco Smoke Carcinogens and Lung Cancer," *J Natl Cancer Inst* 1999; 91: 1194-1210.

Djordjevic, M.V. et al. "Doses of nicotine and lung carcinogens delivered to cigarette smokers," *J Natl Cancer Inst* 2000; 92: 106-11.

Foucart, S. "Les conspirateurs du tabac," *Le Monde*, 25 février 2012.

https://www6.miami.edu/ethics/jpsl/archives/papers/tobacco.html

Proctor, R.N. *Golden Holocaust: Origins of the Cigarette Catastrophe and the Case for Abolition*, University of California Press, 752 pages, 2012.

Kabbani, N. "Not so cool? Menthol's discovered actions on the nicotinic receptor and its implications for nicotine addiction," *Frontiers in Neuropharmacology* 2013; 4: 95.

National Cancer Institute. *Risks Associated With Smoking Cigarettes With Low Machine-Measured Yields of Tar and Nicotine*, Smoking and Tobacco Control Monograph No. 13, U.S. Department of Health and Human Services, National Institutes of Health, National Cancer Institute, NIH Publication No. 02-5074.

Ng, M. et al. "Smoking prevalence and cigarette consumption in 187 countries 1980-2012," *JAMA* 2014; 311: 183-92. www.legacy.library.ucsf.edu

Pleasance, E.D. et al. "A small-cell lung cancer genome with complex signatures of tobacco exposure," *Nature* 2010; 463: 184-190.

www.epa.gov/radiation/sources/tobacco.html

Proctor, R.N. "Puffing on Polonium," *The New York Times*, 1er décembre 2006.

Rego, B. *The Polonium Brief. A Hidden History of Cancer, Radiation, and the Tobacco Industry*, Isis 2009; 100: 453-84.

Besaratinia, A. et S. Tommasi. "Genotoxicity of tobacco smoke-derived aromatic amines and bladder cancer: current state of knowledge and future research directions," *FASEB J* 2013; 27: 2090-2100.

Alberg, A.J. et J.R. Hébert. "Cigarette smoking and bladder cancer: a new twist in an old saga?," *J Natl Cancer Inst* 2009; 101: 1525-1526.

Doll, R. et al. "Mortality in relation to smoking: 50 years' observations on male British doctors," *BMJ* 2004; 328: 1519.

Ng, M. et al. "Smoking prevalence and cigarette consumption in 187 countries 1980-2012," *JAMA* 2014; 311: 183-92.

Smith, A.L. et S. Chapman. "Quitting smoking unassisted: the 50-year research neglect of a major public health phenomenon," *JAMA* 2014; 311: 137-8.

Stead, L.F. et al. "Nicotine replacement therapy for smoking cessation," *Cochrane Database Syst Rev* 2012; 11: CD000146.

Mons, U. et al. "Impact of national smoke-free legislation on home smoking bans: findings from the International Tobacco Control Policy Evaluation Project Europe Surveys," *Tob Control* 2013; 22: e2-9.

www.nytimes.com/1993/11/28/opinion/in-america-tobacco-dollars.html

Fairchild, A.L. et al. "The renormalization of smoking? E-cigarettes and the tobacco "endgame"," *N Engl J Med* 2014; 370: 293-5.

Dawkins, L. et al. ""Vaping" profiles and preferences: an online survey of electronic cigarette users," *Addiction* 2013; 108: 1115-25.

Sweanor, D. et al. "Tobacco harm reduction: how rational public policy could transform a pandemic," *Int J Drug Policy* 2007; 18: 70-4.

Grana, R. et al. "E-cigarettes: a scientific review," *Circulation* 2014; 129: 1972-86.

Brown, J. et al. "Real-world effectiveness of e-cigarettes when used to aid smoking cessation: a cross-sectional population study," *Addiction* 2014 May 20. doi: 10.1111/add.12623. [Epub avant publication].

Chapter 3

Stuckler, D. et M. Nestle. "Big food, food systems, and global health," *PLoS Med* 2012; 9: e1001242.

Moss, M. *Salt Sugar Fat: How the Food Giants Hooked Us*, Random House, 480 pages, 2013.

Blumenthal, D.M. et M.S. Gold. "Neurobiology of food addiction," *Curr Opin Clin Nutr Metab Care* 2010; 13: 359-65.

Volkow, N.D. et al. "Overlapping neuronal circuits in addiction and obesity: evidence of systems pathology," *Philos Trans R Soc Lond B Biol Sci* 2008; 363: 3191-3200.

Lenoir, M. et al. "Intense sweetness surpasses cocaine reward," *PLoS One* 2007; 2(8): e698.

Johnson, P.M. et P.J. Kenny. "Dopamine D2 receptors in addiction-like reward dysfunction and compulsive eating in obese rats," *Nat Neurosci* 2010; 13: 635-41.

Burger, K.S. et E. Stice. "Frequent ice cream consumption is associated with reduced striatal response to receipt of an ice cream-based milkshake," *Am J Clin Nutr* 2012; 95: 810-7.

Gearhardt, A.N. et al. "The addiction potential of hyperpalatable foods," *Curr Drug Abuse Rev* 2011; 4: 140-5.

Ziauddeen, H. et al. "Obesity and the brain: how convincing is the addiction model?," *Nat Rev Neurosci* 2012; 13: 279-86.

Guyenet, S.J. "Seduced by Food: Obesity and the Human Brain" (http://boingboing.net/2012/03/09/seduced-by-food-obesity-and-t.html)

Westerterp, K.R. et J.R. Speakman. "Physical activity energy expenditure has not declined since the 1980s and matches energy expenditure of wild animals," *Int J Obes* 2008; 32: 1256-63.

Swinburn, B. et al. "Increased food energy supply is more than sufficient to explain the US epidemic of obesity," *Am J Clin Nutr* 2009; 90: 1453-6.

http://win.niddk.nih.gov/publications/PDFs/stat904z.pdf

Stuckler, D. et al. "Manufacturing epidemics: the role of global producers in increased consumption of unhealthy commodities including processed foods, alcohol, and tobacco," *PLoS Med* 2012; 9: e1001235.

Doak, C. et al. "Overweight and underweight coexist within households in Brazil, China and Russia," *J Nutr* 2000; 130: 2965-2971.

Wellen, K.E. et G.S. Hotamisligil. "Inflammation, stress, and diabetes," *J Clin Invest* 2005; 115: 1111-9.

Taube, A. et al. "Inflammation and metabolic dysfunction: links to cardiovascular diseases," *Am J Physiol Heart Circ Physiol* 2012; 302: H2148-65.

Prospective Studies Collaboration, G. Whitlock, S. Lewington, P. Sherliker et al. "Body-mass index and cause-specific mortality in 900 000 adults: collaborative analyses of 57 prospective studies," *Lancet* 2009; 373 (9669): 1083-1096.

http://rhumatologie.edimark.fr/phototheque/galerie_detail.php?id_galerie=2272

Reeves, G.K. et al. "Cancer incidence and mortality in relation to body mass index in the Million Women Study: cohort study," *BMJ* 2007; 335: 1134-1200.

Renehan, A. et al. "Body mass index and incidence of cancer: a systematic review and meta-analysis of prospective observational studies," *Lancet* 2008; 371: 569-578.

Manson, J.E. et al. "Body weight and mortality among women," *New Engl J Med* 1995; 333: 677-685.

Khandekar, M.J. et al. "Molecular mechanisms of cancer development in obesity," *Nat Rev Cancer* 2011; 11: 886-95.

Williams, S.C.P. "Link between obesity and cancer," *Proc Natl Acad Sci USA* 2013; 110: 8753-54.

Campbell, P.T. et al. "Excess body weight and colorectal cancer risk in Canada: associations in subgroups of clinically defined familial risk of cancer," *Cancer Epidemiol Biomarkers Prev* 2007; 16: 1735-1744.

Yun, K.E. et al. "Impact of body mass index on the risk of colorectal adenoma in a metabolically healthy population," *Cancer Res* 2013; 73: 4020-7.

Nock, N.L. et N.A. Berger. "Obesity and cancer: overview of mechanisms," Berger N.A. (ed.) *Cancer and Energy Balance, Epidemiology and Overview*, Springer, 2010: 129-179.

Cohen, D.H. et D. LeRoith. "Obesity, type 2 diabetes, and cancer: the insulin and IGF connection," *Endocr Relat Cancer* 2012; 19: F27-45.

Attner, B. et al. "Cancer among patients with diabetes and abnormal blood lipids: a population based register study in Sweden," *Cancer Causes Control* 2012; 23: 769-777.

Hirakawa, Y. et al. "Association between glucose tolerance level and cancer death in a general Japanese population: the Hisayama Study," *Am J Epidemiol* 2012; 176: 856-64.

www.nytimes.com/2013/05/19/magazine/say-hello-to-the-100-trillion-bacteria-that-make-up-your-microbiome.html?pagewanted=all

Kessler, D.A. *The End of Overeating: Taking Control of the Insatiable American Appetite*, New York, Rodale Books, 2010.

Ahn, J. et al. "Human gut microbiome and risk for colorectal cancer," *J Natl Cancer Inst* 2013; 105: 1907-11.

Yoshimoto, S. et al. "Obesity-induced gut microbial metabolite promotes liver cancer through senescence secretome," *Nature* 2013; 499: 97-101.

Turnbaugh, P.J. et al. "A core gut microbiome in obese and lean twins," *Nature* 2009; 457: 480-4.

Pollan, M. "Some of My Best Friends Are Germs," *The New York Times Magazine*, 15 mai 2013.

David, L.A. et al. "Diet rapidly and reproducibly alters the human gut microbiome," *Nature* 2014; 505: 559-63.

www.iarc.fr/en/publications/books/wcr/

Stuckler, D. et al. "Manufacturing epidemics: the role of global producers in increased consumption of unhealthy commodities including processed foods, alcohol, and tobacco," *PLoS Med* 2012; 9: e1001235.

Brownell, K.D. et K.E. Warner. "The perils of ignoring history: Big Tobacco played dirty and millions died. How similar is Big Food?," *Milbank Q* 2009; 87: 259-94.

Pereira, M.A. et al. "Fast-food habits, weight gain, and insulin resistance (the CARDIA study): 15-year prospective analysis," *Lancet* 2005; 365: 36-42.

Hu, F.B. et V.S. Malik. "Sugar-sweetened beverages and risk of obesity and type 2 diabetes: epidemiologic evidence," *Physiol Behav* 2010; 100: 47-54.

Moreno, L. et G. Rodriguez. "Dietary risk factors for development of childhood obesity," *Curr Opin Clin Nutr Metab Care* 2007; 10: 336-341.

http://eming.com/en/life-expectancy-of-okinawan-is-shortening-who-is-the-culprit-fast-food/

www.nytimes.com/2008/09/24/world/europe/24diet.html?pagewanted=all&_r=0

Stewart, S.T. et al. "Forecasting the effects of obesity and smoking on U.S. life expectancy," *N Engl J Med* 2009; 361: 2252-60.

Jolliffe, D. "Extent of overweight among US children and adolescents from 1971 to 2000," *Int J Obes Relat Metab Disord* 2004; 28: 4-9.

Cunningham, S.A. et al. "Incidence of childhood obesity in the United States," *N Engl J Med* 2014; 370: 403-11.

Malik, V.S. et al. "Sugar-sweetened beverages and risk of metabolic syndrome and type 2 diabetes: a meta-analysis," *Diabetes Care* 2010; 33: 2477-2483.

Lustig, R.H. et al. "Public health: the toxic truth about sugar," *Nature* 2012; 482: 27-9.

Bray, G.A. et B.M. Popkin. "Dietary sugar and body weight: have we reached a crisis in the epidemic of obesity and diabetes? Health be damned! Pour on the sugar," *Diabetes Care* 2014; 37: 950-6.

Swithers, S.E. "Artificial sweeteners produce the counterintuitive effect of inducing metabolic derangements," *Trends Endocrinol Metab* 2013; 24: 431-41.

Dhingra, R. et al. "Soft drink consumption and risk of developing cardiometabolic risk factors and the metabolic syndrome in middle-aged adults in the community," *Circulation* 2007; 116: 480-8.

Giovannucci, E. et al. "Diabetes and cancer: a consensus report," *Diabetes Care* 2010; 33:1674-85.

Chapter 4

http://chrisagde.free.fr/bourb/l14vie.php3?page=38

"Aroma compounds," *Food Chemistry* 2009: 340-402.

Brewer, M.S. *The Chemistry of Beef Flavor – Executive Summary*, National Cattlemen's Beef Association, 2006.

www.iol.co.za/lifestyle/food-drink/food/why-does-meat-taste-so-good-1.1568195#.UijfehbiOXo

Fonseca-Azevedo, K. et S. Herculano-Houzel. "Metabolic constraint imposes tradeoff between body size and number of brain neurons in human evolution," *Proc Natl Acad Sci USA* 2012; 109: 18571-6.

Gorman, R.M. "Cooking Up Bigger Brains," *Scientific American*, 16 décembre 2007.

Psouni, E. et al. "Impact of carnivory on human development and evolution revealed by a new unifying model of weaning in mammals," *PLoS One* 2012; 7: e32452.

Zeder, M.A. "Domestication and early agriculture in the Mediterranean Basin: Origins, diffusion, and impact," *Proc Natl Acad Sci USA* 2008; 105: 11597-11604.

Storey, A.A. et al. "Investigating the global dispersal of chickens in prehistory using ancient mitochondrial DNA signatures," *PLoS One* 2012; 7: e39171.

Robitaille, J. "La consommation de viande : Évolution et perspectives de croissance," *BioClips* + 2012; 15: 1-12.

www.passeportsante.net/documentsproteus/popuphtml/hypercholesterolemie_tableaux.htm

www.editions-homme.com/gibier/PDF/tendrete.pdf

www.todayifoundout.com/index.php/2010/04/the-red-juice-in-raw-red-meat-is-not-blood/

www.blackpudding.org/history/

http://russelleaton.articlealley.com/numbers-of-vegetarians-are-growing-world-wide-1351542.html

www.who.int/nutrition/topics/3_foodconsumption/en/index4.html

Globocan 2008. http://www-dep.iarc.fr

Kuriki, K. and K. Tajima. "The increasing incidence of colorectal cancer and the preventive strategy in Japan," *Asian Pacific J Cancer Prev* 2006; 7: 495-501.

Daniel, C.R. et al. "Prospective investigation of poultry and fish intake in relation to cancer risk," *Cancer Prev Res (Phila)* 2011; 4: 1903-11.

Chan, D.S. et al. "Red and processed meat and colorectal cancer incidence: meta-analysis of prospective studies," *PLoS One* 2011; 6: e20456.

Pan, A. et al. "Red meat consumption and mortality: results from 2 prospective cohort studies," *Arch Intern Med* 2012; 172: 555-63.

Rohrmann, S. et al. "Meat consumption and mortality: results from the European Prospective Investigation into Cancer and Nutrition," *BMC Medicine* 2013; 11: 63.

Sinha, R. et al. "Meat intake and mortality: a prospective study of over half a million people," *Arch Intern Med* 2009; 169: 562-71.

Pan, A. et al. "Red meat consumption and risk of type 2 diabetes: 3 cohorts of US adults and an updated meta-analysis," *Am J Clin Nutr* 2011; 94(4): 1088-1096.

Tappel, A. "Heme of consumed red meat can act as a catalyst of oxidative damage and could initiate colon, breast and prostate cancers, heart disease and other diseases," *Med Hypotheses* 2007; 68: 562-4.

Cross, A.J. et al. "Haem, not protein or inorganic iron, is responsible for endogenous intestinal N-nitrosation arising from red meat," *Cancer Res* 2003; 63: 2358-60.

Jakszyn, P. et al. "Development of a food database of nitrosamines, heterocyclic amines, and polycyclic aromatic hydrocarbons," *J Nutr* 2004; 134: 2011-14.

Cross, A.J. et al. "A prospective study of red and processed meat intake in relation to cancer risk," *PLoS Med* 2007; 4: e325.

De Stefani, E. et al. "Processed meat consumption and risk of cancer: a multisite case-control study in Uruguay," *Br J Cancer* 2012; 107: 1584-8.

www.precisionnutrition.com/all-about-cooking-carcinogens

Cross, A.J. et al. "A large prospective study of meat consumption and colorectal cancer risk: an investigation of potential mechanisms underlying this association," *Cancer Res* 2010; 70: 2406-2414.

Stolzenberg-Solomon, R.Z. et al. "Meat and meat-mutagen intake and pancreatic cancer risk in the NIH-AARP cohort," *Cancer Epidemiol Biomarkers Prevention* 2007; 16: 2664-2675.

Sinha, R. et al. "Meat and meat-related compounds and risk of prostate cancer in a large prospective cohort study in the United States," *Am J Epidemiol* 2009; 170: 1165-1177.

Puangsombat, K. et al. "Occurrence of heterocyclic amines in cooked meat products," *Meat Sci* 2012; 90: 739-46.

Viegas, O. et al. "Inhibitory effect of antioxidant-rich marinades on the formation of heterocyclic aromatic amines in pan-fried beef," *J Agric Food Chem* 2012; 60: 6235-40.

Gibis, M. and J. Weiss. "Antioxidant capacity and inhibitory effect of grape seed and rosemary extract in marinades on the formation of heterocyclic amines in fried beef patties," *Food Chem* 2012; 134: 766-74.

Li, Z. et al. "Antioxidant-rich spice added to hamburger meat during cooking results in reduced meat, plasma, and urine malondialdehyde concentrations," *Am J Clin Nutr* 2010; 91: 1180-4.

Nerurkar, P.V. et al. "Effects of marinating with Asian marinades or western barbecue sauce on PhIP and MeIQx formation in barbecued beef," *Nutr Cancer* 1999; 34: 147-52.

Puangsombat, K. et al. "Inhibitory activity of Asian spices on heterocyclic amines formation in cooked beef patties," *J Food Sci* 2011; 76: T174-80.

Salmon, C.P. et al. "Effects of marinating on heterocyclic amine carcinogen formation in grilled chicken," *Food Chem Toxicol* 1997; 35: 433-41.

Romero, S. "Argentina Falls From Its Throne as King of Beef," *The New York Times*, 13 June 2013.

Miller, G.J. "Lipids in wild ruminant animals and steers," *J of Food Quality* 1986; 9: 331-343.

Parasramka, M.A. et al. "MicroRNA profiling of carcinogen-induced rat colon tumors and the influence of dietary spinach," *Mol Nutr Food Res* 2012; 56: 1259-69.

De Vogel, J. et al. "Green vegetables, red meat and colon cancer: chlorophyll prevents the cytotoxic and hyperproliferative effects of haem in rat colon," *Carcinogenesis* 2005; 26: 387-93.

Klein, E. "Taking antibiotics you don't really need might kill you," *The Washington Post*, 16 septembre 2013 (www.washingtonpost.com/blogs/wonkblog/wp/2013/09/16/taking-antibiotics-you-dont-really-need-might-kill-you/).

Allan, N. "We're running out of antibiotics," *The Atlantic*, mars 2014, p. 34.

www.pewhealth.org/other-resource/record-high-antibiotic-sales-for-meat-and-poultry-production-85899449119

Levine, M.E. et al. "Low protein intake is associated with a major reduction in IGF-1, cancer, and overall mortality in the 65 and younger but not older population," *Cell Metabolism* 2014; 19: 407-417.

Chapter 5

Monteiro, C.A. and G. Cannon. "The impact of transnational "big food" companies on the South: a view from Brazil," *PLoS Med* 2012; 9: e1001252.

Centers for Disease Control and Prevention. State-Specific Trends in Fruit and Vegetable Consumption among Adults - United States, 2000-2009, *MMWR* 2010; 59: 1125-1130.

Kimmons, J. et al. "Fruit and vegetable intake among adolescents and adults in the United States: percentage meeting individualized recommendations," *Medscape J Med* 2009; 11: 26.

Hall, J.N. et al. "Global variability in fruit and vegetable consumption," *Am J Prev Med* 2009; 36: 402-409.

www.ers.usda.gov/data-products/chart-gallery/detail.aspx?chartId=40452#.Ut6D4nnq7-Y

www.ars.usda.gov/main/site_main.htm?modecode=12-35-45-00

Mori, K. et al. "Fucoxanthin and its metabolites in edible brown algae cultivated in deep seawater," *Mar Drugs* 2004; 2: 63-72.

Hung, H.C. et al. "Fruit and vegetable intake and risk of major chronic disease," *J Natl Cancer Inst* 2004; 96: 1577-84.

Bhupathiraju, S.N. et al. "Quantity and variety in fruit and vegetable intake and risk of coronary heart disease," *Am J Clin Nutr* 2013; 98: 1514-23.

Boffetta, P. et al. "Fruit and vegetable intake and overall cancer risk in the European Prospective Investigation into Cancer and Nutrition (EPIC)," *J Natl Cancer Inst* 2010; 102: 529-37.

Michaud, D.S. et al. "Fruit and vegetable intake and incidence of bladder cancer in a male prospective cohort," *J Natl Cancer Inst* 1999; 91: 605-13.

Wu, Q.J. et al. "Cruciferous vegetables consumption and the risk of female lung cancer: a prospective study and a meta-analysis," *Ann Oncol* 2013; 24: 1918-24.

Masala, G. et al. "Fruit and vegetables consumption and breast cancer risk: the EPIC Italy study," *Breast Cancer Res Treat* 2012; 132: 1127-36.

Yang, G. et al. "Prospective cohort study of green tea consumption and colorectal cancer risk in women," *Cancer Epidemiol Biomarkers Prev* 2007; Jun 16(6): 1219-23.

Gonzalez, C.A. et al. "Fruit and vegetable intake and the risk of gastric adenocarcinoma: a reanalysis of the European Prospective Investigation into Cancer and Nutrition (EPIC-EURGAST) study after a longer follow-up," *Int J Cancer* 2012; 131: 2910-9.

Fung, T.T. et al. "Intake of specific fruits and vegetables in relation to risk of estrogen receptor-negative breast cancer among postmenopausal women," *Breast Cancer Res Treat* 2013; 138: 925-30.

Bao, Y. et al. "Nut consumption and risk of pancreatic cancer in women," *Br J Cancer* 2013; 109: 2911-6.

Lock, K. et al. "Low fruit and vegetable consumption," I.M. Ezzati, A.D. Lopez, A. Rodgers, C.J.L. Murray, , dir. *Comparative quantification of health risks: global and regional burden of disease attributable to selected major risk factors*, Genève, WHO, 2004.

Bellavia, A. et al. "Fruit and vegetable consumption and all-cause mortality: a dose-response analysis," *Am J Clin Nutr* 2013; 98: 454-9.

Zamora-Ros, R. et al. "High concentrations of a urinary biomarker of polyphenol intake are associated with decreased mortality in older adults," *J Nutr* 2013; 143: 1445-50.

Lam, T.K. et al. "Cruciferous vegetable intake and lung cancer risk: a nested case-control study matched on cigarette smoking," *Cancer Epidemiol Biomarkers Prev* 2010; 19: 2534-40.

Michaud, D.S. et al. "Fruit and vegetable intake and incidence of bladder cancer in a male prospective cohort," *J Natl Cancer Inst* 1999; 91: 605-13.

Watson, G.W. et al. "Phytochemicals from cruciferous vegetables, epigenetics, and prostate cancer prevention," *AAPS J* 2013; 15: 951-61.

Tse, G. and G.D. Eslick. "Cruciferous vegetables and risk of colorectal neoplasms: a systematic review and meta-analysis," *Nutr Cancer* 2014; 66: 128-39.

Wu, Q.J. et al. "Cruciferous vegetable consumption and gastric cancer risk: a meta-analysis of epidemiological studies," *Cancer Sci* 2013; 104: 1067-73.

Suzuki, R. et al. "Fruit and vegetable intake and breast cancer risk defined by estrogen and progesterone receptor status: the Japan Public Health Center-based Prospective Study," *Cancer Causes Control* 2013; 24: 2117-28.

Zhang, C.X. et al. "Greater vegetable and fruit intake is associated with a lower risk of breast cancer among Chinese women," *Int J Cancer* 2009; 125: 181-188.

Bosetti, C. et al. "Cruciferous vegetables and cancer risk in a network of case-control studies," *Ann Oncol* 2012; 23: 2198-203.

International Agency for Research on Cancer. *IARC Handbooks of Cancer Prevention Volume 9 Cruciferous vegetables, Isothiocyanates and Indoles*, Lyon, IARC Press, 2004.

Dosz, E.B. et E.H. Jeffery. "Modifying the processing and handling of frozen broccoli for increased sulforaphane formation," *J Food Sci* 2013; 78: H1459-63.

Rivlin, R.S. "Historical perspective on the use of garlic," *J Nutr* 2001; 131: 951S-4S.

Gonzalez, C.A. et al. "Fruit and vegetable intake and the risk of stomach and oesophagus adenocarcinoma in the European Prospective Investigation into Cancer and Nutrition (EPIC-EURGAST)," *Int J Cancer* 2006; 118: 2559-2566.

Gao, C.M. et al. "Protective effect of allium vegetables against both esophageal and stomach cancer: a simultaneous case-referent study of a high-epidemic area in Jiangsu Province, China," *Jap J Cancer Res* 1999; 90: 614-621.

Steinmetz, K.A. et al. "Vegetables, fruit, and colon cancer in the Iowa Women's Health Study," *Am J of Epidemiol* 1994; 139: 1-15.

Hsing, A.W. et al. "Allium vegetables and risk of prostate cancer: a population-based study," *J Natl Cancer Inst* 2002; 94: 1648-1651.

Chan, J.M. et al. "Vegetable and fruit intake and pancreatic cancer in a population-based case-control study in the San Francisco bay area," *Cancer Epidemiol Biomarkers Prev* 2005; 14: 2093-2097.

Challier, B. et al. "Garlic, onion and cereal fibre as protective factors for breast cancer: a French case-control study," *Eur J Epidemiol* 1998; 14: 737-747.

Milner, J.A. "A historical perspective on garlic and cancer," *J Nutr* 2001; 131: 1027S-31S.

www.cancer.gov/cancertopics/factsheet/prevention/garlic-and-cancer-prevention

Wu, K. et al. "Plasma and dietary carotenoids, and the risk of prostate cancer: a nested case-control study," *Cancer Epidemiol Biomarkers Prev* 2004; 13: 260-9.

Zhang, X. et al. "Carotenoid intakes and risk of breast cancer defined by estrogen receptor and progesterone receptor status: a pooled analysis of 18 prospective cohort studies," *Am J Clin Nutr* 2012; 95: 713-25.

Michaud, D.S. et al. "Intake of specific carotenoids and risk of lung cancer in 2 prospective US cohorts," *Am J Clin Nutr* 2000; 72: 990-997.

Le Marchand, L. et al. "An ecological study of diet and lung cancer in the South Pacific," *Int J Cancer* 1995; 63: 18-23.

Kumar, S.R. et al. "Fucoxanthin: a marine carotenoid exerting anti-cancer effects by affecting multiple mechanisms," *Mar Drugs* 2013; 11: 5130-5147.

Sho, H. "History and characteristics of Okinawan longevity food," *Asia Pac J Clin Nutr* 2001; 10(2): 159-64.

Lamy, S. et al. "Delphinidin, a dietary anthocyanidin, inhibits vascular endothelial growth factor receptor-2 phosphorylation," *Carcinogenesis* 2006; 27: 989-96.

Labrecque, L. et al. "Combined inhibition of PDGF and VEGF receptors by ellagic acid, a dietary-derived phenolic compound," *Carcinogenesis* 2005; 26: 821-6.

Adams, L.S. et al. "Blueberry phytochemicals inhibit growth and metastatic potential of MDA-MB-231 breast cancer cells through modulation of the phosphatidylinositol 3-kinase pathway," *Cancer Res* 2010; 70: 3594-3605.

Moghe, S. et al. "Effect of blueberry polyphenols on 3T3-F442A preadipocyte differentiation," *J Med Food* 2012; 15: 448-52.

Prior, R.L. et al. "Purified blueberry anthocyanins and blueberry juice alter development of obesity in mice fed an obesogenic high-fat diet," *J Agric Food Chem* 2010; 58: 3970-3976.

Wedick, N.M. et al. "Dietary flavonoid intakes and risk of type 2 diabetes in US men and women," *Am J Clin Nutr* 2012; 95: 925-33.

Brown, E.M. et al. "Persistence of anticancer activity in berry extracts after simulated gastrointestinal digestion and colonic fermentation," *PLoS One* 2012; 7: e49740.

Rababah, T.M. et al. "Effect of jam processing and storage on total phenolics, antioxidant activity, and anthocyanins of different fruits," *J Sci Food Agric* 2011; 91: 1096-102.

Rodriguez-Mateos, A. et al. "Impact of cooking, proving, and baking on the (poly)phenol content of wild blueberry," *J Agric Food Chem*, 2014; 62: 3979-3986.

Yang, C.S. et al. "Cancer prevention by tea: animal studies, molecular mechanisms and human relevance," *Nat Rev Cancer* 2009; 9: 429-39.

Nechuta, S. et al. "Prospective cohort study of tea consumption and risk of digestive system cancers: results from the Shanghai Women's Health Study," *Am J Clin Nutr* 2012; 96: 1056-63.

Tang, N. et al. "Green tea, black tea consumption and risk of lung cancer: a meta-analysis," *Lung Cancer* 2009; 65: 274-83.

Kurahashi, N. et al. "Green tea consumption and prostate cancer risk in Japanese men: a prospective study," *Am J Epidemiol* 2008; 167: 71-7.

Zhang, M. et al. "Green tea and the prevention of breast cancer: a case-control study in Southeast China," *Carcinogenesis* 2007; 28: 1074-8.

Deandrea, S. et al. "Is temperature an effect modifier of the association between green tea intake and gastric cancer risk?," *Eur J Cancer Prev* 2010; 19: 18-22.

Kurahashi, N. et al. "Plasma isoflavones and subsequent risk of prostate cancer in a nested case-control study: the Japan Public Health Center," *J Clin Oncol* 2008; 26: 5923-9.

Lee, S.A. et al. "Adolescent and adult soy food intake and breast cancer risk: results from the Shanghai Women's Health Study," *Am J Clin Nutr* 2009; 89: 1920-6.

Dong, J.Y. and L.Q. Qin. "Soy isoflavones consumption and risk of breast cancer incidence or recurrence: a meta-analysis of prospective studies," *Breast Cancer Res Treat* 2011; 125: 315-23.

Ollberding, N.J. et al. "Legume, soy, tofu, and isoflavone intake and endometrial cancer risk in postmenopausal women in the multiethnic cohort study," *J Natl Cancer Inst* 2012; 104: 67-76.

Yang, W.S. et al. "Soy intake is associated with lower lung cancer risk: results from a meta-analysis of epidemiologic studies," *Am J Clin Nutr* 2011; 94: 1575-83.

Taylor, C.K. et al. "The effect of genistein aglycone on cancer and cancer risk: a review of in vitro, preclinical, and clinical studies," *Nutr Rev* 2009; 67: 398-415.

Fritz, H. et al. "Soy, red clover, and isoflavones and breast cancer: a systematic review," *PLoS One* 2013; 8: e81968.

Bao, Y. et al. "Association of nut consumption with total and cause-specific mortality," *N Engl J Med* 2013; 369: 2001-11.

Guasch-Ferré, M. et al. "Frequency of nut consumption and mortality risk in the PREDIMED nutrition intervention trial," *BMC Med* 2013; 11: 164.

Singh, P.N. and G.E. Fraser. "Dietary risk factors for colon cancer in a low-risk population," *Am J Epidemiol* 1998; 148: 761-774.

González, C.A. et J. Salas-Salvadó. "The potential of nuts in the prevention of cancer," *Br J Nutr* 2006; 96 Suppl 2: S87-94.

Bes-Rastrollo, M. et al. "Prospective study of nut consumption, long-term weight change, and obesity risk in women," *Am J Clin Nutr* 2009; 89: 1913-1919.

Berkey, C.S. et al. "Vegetable protein and vegetable fat intakes in pre-adolescent and adolescent girls, and risk for benign breast disease in young women," *Breast Cancer Res Treat* 2013; 141: 299-306.

Demark-Wahnefried, W. et al. "Flaxseed supplementation (not dietary fat restriction) reduces prostate cancer proliferation rates in men presurgery," *Cancer Epidemiol Biomarkers Prev* 2008; 17: 3577-87.

Lowcock, E.C. et al. "Consumption of flaxseed, a rich source of lignans, is associated with reduced breast cancer risk," *Cancer Causes Control* 2013; 24: 813-6.

Buck, K. et al. "Meta-analyses of lignans and enterolignans in relation to breast cancer risk," *Am J Clin Nutr* 2010; 92: 141-153.

Eichholzer, M. et al. "Urinary lignans and inflammatory markers in the US National Health and Nutrition Examination Survey (NHANES) 1999-2004 and 2005-2008," *Cancer Causes Control* 2014; 25: 395-403.

Murphy, N. et al. "Dietary fibre intake and risks of cancers of the colon and rectum in the European prospective investigation into cancer and nutrition (EPIC)," *PLoS One* 2012; 7: e39361.

Steevens, J. et al. "Vegetables and fruits consumption and risk of esophageal and gastric cancer subtypes in the Netherlands Cohort Study," *Int J Cancer* 2011; 129: 2681-93.

Mitrou, P.N. et al. "Mediterranean dietary pattern and prediction of all-cause mortality in a US population: results from the NIH-AARP Diet and Health Study," *Arch Intern Med* 2007; 167: 2461-8.

Beauchamp, G.K. et al. "Phytochemistry: ibuprofen-like activity in extra-virgin olive oil," *Nature* 2005; 437: 45-6.

Johnson, C.C. et al. "Non-steroidal anti-inflammatory drug use and colorectal polyps in the Prostate, Lung, Colorectal, and Ovarian Cancer Screening Trial," *Am J Gastroenterol* 2010; 105: 2646-55.

Lamy, S. et al. "Olive oil compounds inhibit vascular endothelial growth factor receptor-2 phosphorylation," *Exp Cell Res* 2014; 322: 89-98.

Peyrot des Gachons, C. et al. "Unusual pungency from extra-virgin olive oil is attributable to restricted spatial expression of the receptor of oleocanthal," *J Neurosci* 2011; 31: 999-1009.

Chapter 6

http://remacle.org/bloodwolf/erudits/Hippocrate/regime.htm

www.bestday.com/editorial/raramuri-races/

www.goodreads.com/quotes/292670-we-say-the-rarajipari-is-the-game-of-life

Booth, F.W. et al. "Reduced physical activity and risk of chronic disease: the biology behind the consequences," *Eur J Appl Physiol* 2008; 102: 381-390.

Bramble, D.M. et al. "Endurance running and the evolution of Homo," *Nature* 2004; 432: 345-352.

Statistique Canada. *L'activité physique mesurée directement des adultes canadiens, 2007 à 2011* (www.statcan.gc.ca/pub/82-625-x/2013001/article/11807-fra.htm).

Chevalier, R. "Les aléas de la vie de sofa," *La Presse*, 22 mai 2005.

Morris, J.N. et al. "Coronary heart-disease and physical activity of work," *Lancet* 1953; 265: 1053-7.

Naci, H. et J.P.A. Ioannidis. "Comparative effectiveness of exercise and drug interventions on mortality outcomes: metaepidemiological study," *BMJ* 2013; 347: f5577.

Wolin, K.Y. et al. "Physical activity and colon cancer prevention: a meta-analysis," *Br J Cancer* 2009; 100: 611-616.

Lynch, B.M. et al. "Physical activity and breast cancer prevention," *Recent Results Cancer Res* 2011; 186: 13-42.

Arem, H. et al. "Physical activity and cancer-specific mortality in the NIH-AARP Diet and Health Study cohort," *Int J Cancer* 2014; 135: 423-31.

Brown, J.C. et al. "Cancer, physical activity, and exercise," *Compr Physiol* 2012; 2: 2775-809.

Matthews, C.E. et al. "Amount of time spent in sedentary behaviors and cause-specific mortality in US adults," *Am J Clin Nutr* 2012; 95: 437-45.

Lee, I.M. et al. "Effect of physical inactivity on major non-communicable diseases worldwide: an analysis of burden of disease and life expectancy," *Lancet* 2012; 380: 219-29.

Colley, R.C. et al. *Physical activity of Canadian adults: accelerometer results from the 2007 to 2009 Canadian Health Measures Survey* (www.statcan.gc.ca/pub/82-003-x/2011001/article/11396-eng.htm).

Schmid, D. and M. Leitzmann. "Television viewing and time spent sedentary in relation to cancer risk: a meta-analysis," *J Natl Cancer Inst* 2014 doi:10.1093/jnci/dju098.

http://preventcancer.aicr.org/site/News2?page=NewsArticle&id=13891

www.hsph.harvard.edu/obesity-prevention-source/obesity-causes/physical-activity-and-obesity/

www.aicr.org/press/press-releases/getting-up-from-your-desk.html

www.nih.gov/news/health/nov2012/nci-06.htm

Chapter 7

Wiens, F. et al. "Chronic intake of fermented floral nectar by wild treeshrews," *Proc Natl Acad Sci USA* 2008; 105: 10426-31.

Orbach, D.N. et al. "Drinking and flying: does alcohol consumption affect the flight and echolocation performance of phyllostomid bats?," *PLoS One* 2010; 5: e8993.

Shohat-Ophir, G. et al. "Sexual deprivation increases ethanol intake in Drosophila," *Science* 2012; 335: 1351-5.

Benner, S.A. et al. "Planetary biology-paleontological, geological, and molecular histories of life," *Science* 2002; 296: 864-8.

Benner, S. "Paleogenetics and the history of alcohol in primates," rencontre annuelle de l'American Association for the Advancement of Science (AAAS), Boston, 15 février 2013.

Di Castelnuovo, A. et al. "Alcohol dosing and total mortality in men and women: an updated meta-analysis of 34 prospective studies," *Arch Intern Med* 2006; 166: 2437-45.

Szmitko, P.E. and S. Verma. "Red wine and your heart," *Circulation* 2005; 111: e10-e11.

Opie, L.H. and S. Lecour. "The red wine hypothesis: from concepts to protective signalling molecules," *Eur Heart J* 2007; 28: 1683-93.

Grønbæk, M. et al. "Type of alcohol consumed and mortality from all causes, coronary heart disease, and cancer," *Ann Intern Med* 2000; 133: 411-9.

Klatsky, A.L. et al. "Wine, liquor, beer, and mortality," *Am J Epidemiol* 2003; 158: 585-595.

Renaud, S.C. et al. "Wine, beer, and mortality in middle-aged men from eastern France," *Arch Intern Med* 1999; 159: 1865-1870.

Waterhouse, A.L. "Wine phenolics," *Ann NY Acad Sci* 2002; 957: 21-36.

Yu, W. et al. "Cellular and molecular effects of resveratrol in health and disease," *J Cell Biochem* 2012; 113: 752-759.

Ely, M. "Gender differences in the relationship between alcohol consumption and drink problems are largely accounted for by body water," *Alcohol* 1999; 34: 894-902.

Frezza, M. et al. "High blood alcohol levels in women. The role of decreased gastric alcohol dehydrogenase activity and first-pass metabolism," *N Engl J Med* 1990; 322: 95-9.

www.ccsa.ca/Ressource%20Library/CCSA-Patterns-Alcohol-Use-Policy-Canada-2012-fr.pdf

Liu, Y. et al. "Alcohol intake between menarche and first pregnancy: a prospective study of breast cancer risk," *J Natl Cancer Inst* 2013; 105: 1571-8.

Sundell, L. et al. "Increased stroke risk is related to a binge-drinking habit," *Stroke* 2008; 39: 3179-84.

http://hamsnetwork.org/metabolism/

Peng, Y. et al. "The ADH1B Arg47His polymorphism in east Asian populations and expansion of rice domestication in history," *BMC Evol Biol* 2010; 10: 15.

Brooks, P. et al. "The alcohol flushing response: an unrecognized risk factor for esophageal cancer from alcohol consumption," *PLoS Med* 2009; 6: e50.

Baan, R. et al. "Carcinogenicity of alcoholic beverages," *Lancet Oncol* 2007; 8: 292-3.

Zhang, G. et al. "ADH1B Arg47His polymorphism is associated with esophageal cancer risk in high-incidence Asian populations: evidence from a meta-analysis," *PLoS One* 2010; 5: e13679.

Homann, N. et al. "Increased salivary acetaldehyde levels in heavy drinkers and smokers: a microbiological approach to oral cavity cancer," *Carcinogenesis* 2000; 21: 663-8.

Salaspuro, V. and M. Salaspuro. "Synergistic effect of alcohol drinking and smoking on *in vivo* acetaldehyde concentration in saliva," *Int J Cancer* 2004; 111: 480-3.

Castellsagué, X. et al. "The role of type of tobacco and type of alcoholic beverage in oral carcinogenesis," *Int J Cancer* 2004; 108: 741-9.

Ahrens, W. et al. "Oral health, dental care and mouthwash associated with upper aerodigestive tract cancer risk in Europe: The ARCAGE Study," *Oral Oncol* 2014; 50: 616-25.

Linderborg, K. et al. "A single sip of a strong alcoholic beverage causes exposure to carcinogenic concentrations of acetaldehyde in the oral cavity," *Food Chem Toxicol* 2011; 49: 2103-2106.

Linderborg, K. et al. "Potential mechanism for Calvados-related œsophageal cancer," *Food Chem Toxicol* 2008; 46: 476-479.

Yokoyama, A. et al. "Salivary acetaldehyde concentration according to alcoholic beverage consumed and aldehyde dehydrogenase-2 genotype," *Alcohol Clin Exp Res* 2008; 32: 1607-14.

Allen, N.E. et al. "Moderate alcohol intake and cancer incidence in women," *J Natl Cancer Inst* 2009; 101: 296-305.

Chao, C. "Associations between beer, wine, and liquor consumption and lung cancer: a meta-analysis," *Cancer Epidemiol Biomarkers Prev* 2007; 16: 2436-47.

Benedetti, A. et al. "Lifetime consumption of alcoholic beverages and risk of 13 types of cancer in men: results from a case-control study in Montreal," *Cancer Detect Prev* 2009; 32: 352-62.

Jang, M. et al. "Cancer chemopreventive activity of resveratrol, a natural product derived from grapes," *Science* 1997; 275: 218-20.

Kraft, T.E. et al. "Fighting cancer with red wine? Molecular mechanisms of resveratrol," *Crit Rev Food Sci Nutr* 2009; 49: 782-99.

Subramanian, L. et al. "Resveratrol: Challenges in translation to the clinic – A critical discussion," *Clin Cancer Res* 2010; 16, 5942-5948.

Patel, K.R. et al. "Sulfate metabolites provide an intracellular pool for resveratrol generation and induce autophagy with senescence," *Sci Transl Med* 2013; 5: 205ra133.

Goldberg, D.M. et al. "A global survey of trans-resveratrol concentrations in commercial wines," *Am J Enol Vitic* 1995; 46: 159-165.

Bessaoud, F. and J.-P. Daurès. "Patterns of alcohol (especially wine) consumption and breast cancer risk: a case-control study among a population in Southern France," *Ann Epidemiol* 2008; 18: 467-75.

Dennis, J. et al. "Alcohol consumption and the risk of breast cancer among BRCA1 and BRCA2 mutation carriers," *Breast* 2010; 19: 479-483.

www.who.int/substance_abuse/publications/global_alcohol_report/profiles/en/

Globocan 2012. *Estimated cancer incidence, mortality and prevalence worldwide in 2012.* (http://globocan.iarc.fr).

www.cancer.gov/cancertopics/factsheet/detection/probability-breast-cancer

www.medicinenet.com/script/main/art.asp?articlekey=11014

Chapter 8

Freedman, P. *Out of the East: Spices and the Medieval Imagination*, New Haven, Yale University Press, 2008.

http://education.jlab.org/glossary/abund_ele.html

University of Wisconsin-Madison (14 octobre 2007). "Why Is The Ocean Salty?," *ScienceDaily*, consulté le 21 octobre 2013 (www.sciencedaily.com releases/2007/10/071012104955.htm).

DasSarma, S. and P. DasSarma. "Halophiles," in *eLS*, Chichester, John Wiley & Sons, Ltd, 2012; doi: 10.1002/9780470015902.a0000394.

Joossens, J.V. et al. "Dietary salt, nitrate and stomach cancer mortality in 24 countries. European Cancer Prevention (ECP) and the INTERSALT Cooperative Research Group," *Int J Epidemiol* 1996; 25: 494-504.

International Agency for Research on Cancer. "Schistosomes, Liver Flukes, and *Helicobacter pylori*," *IARC Monographs on the Evaluation of the Carcinogenic Risks to Humans*, 61, Lyon, IARC, 1994.

Linz, B. et al. "An African origin for the intimate association between humans and *Helicobacter pylori*," *Nature* 2007; 445: 915-8.

Kodaman, N. et al. "Human and *Helicobacter pylori* coevolution shapes the risk of gastric disease," *Proc Natl Acad Sci USA* 2014; 111: 1455-60.

Gaddy, J.A. et al. "High dietary salt intake exacerbates *Helicobacter pylori*-induced gastric carcinogenesis," *Infect Immun* 2013; 81: 2258-67.

Kono, S. and Hirohata T. "Nutrition and stomach cancer," *Cancer Causes Control* 1996; 7: 41-55.

Tannenbaum, S.R. et al. "Inhibition of nitrosamine formation by ascorbic acid," *Am J Clin Nutr* 1991; 53: 247S-250S.

Drake, I.M. et al. "Ascorbic acid may protect against human gastric cancer by scavenging mucosal oxygen radicals," *Carcinogenesis* 1996; 17: 559-562.

Fahey, J.W. et al. "Sulforaphane inhibits extracellular, intracellular, and antibiotic-resistant strains of *Helicobacter pylori* and prevents benzo[a]pyrene-induced stomach tumors," *Proc Natl Acad Sci USA* 2002; 99: 7610-5.

Yanaka, A. et al. "Dietary sulforaphane-rich broccoli sprouts reduce colonization and attenuate gastritis in *Helicobacter pylori*-infected mice and humans," *Cancer Prev Res* 2009; 2: 353-60.

Sifferlin, A. "Salty Truth: Adults Worldwide Eating Too Much Sodium," *TIME*, 22 mars 2013.

http://newsroom.heart.org/news/eating-too-much-salt-led-to-nearly-2-3-million-heart-related-deaths-worldwide-in-2010

Kleinewietfeld, M. et al. "Sodium chloride drives autoimmune disease by the induction of pathogenic TH17 cells," *Nature* 2013; 496: 518-22.

Jacobson, M.F. et al. "Changes in sodium levels in processed and restaurant foods, 2005 to 2011," *JAMA Intern Med* 2013; 173: 1285-1291.

www.newscientist.com/article/dn24086-spicy-food-on-the-menu-6000-years-ago.html#.UlgT6RbiOXo

Saul, H. et al. "Phytoliths in pottery reveal the use of spice in European prehistoric cuisine," *PLoS One* 2013; 8: e70583.

Billing, J. and P.W. Sherman. "Antimicrobial functions of spices: why some like it hot," *Q Rev Biol* 1998; 73: 3-49.

Sherman, P.W. and J. Billing. "Darwinian gastronomy: why we use spices," *Bioscience* 1999; 49: 453-463.

Silva, F. et al. "Coriander (*Coriandrum sativum L.*) essential oil: its antibacterial activity and mode of action evaluated by flow cytometry," *J Med Microbiol* 2011; 60: 1479-1486.

National Nutrition Monitoring Bureau. *NNMB-Annual Reports.* National Institute of Nutrition, Indian Council of Medical Research, Hyderabad, Inde (www.nnmbindia.org/NNMB-PDF%20FILES/Report_for_the_year_1981.pdf).

www.spicehistory.net/spice%20consumption%20data.html

"Spices and Herbs: A survey of the Netherlands and other major markets in the European union" (www.faoda.org/download/Spices_and_Herbs_Survey.pdf).

Globocan 2008. "Estimated Cancer Incidence, Mortality, Prevalence and Disability-adjusted Life Years (DALYs) Worldwide in 2008" (http://globocan.iarc.fr).

Ferlay, J. et al. "Cancer incidence and mortality patterns in Europe: Estimates for 40 countries in 2012," *Eur J Cancer* 2013; 49: 1374-1403.

Aggarwal, B.B. et al. "Molecular targets of nutraceuticals derived from dietary spices: potential role in suppression of inflammation and tumorigenesis," *Exp Biol Med* 2009; 234: 825-49.

Kashyap, A. and S. Weber. "Harappan plant use revealed by starch grains from Farmana, India," *Antiquity* 2010; 84 (http://antiquity.ac.uk/projgall/kashyap326/).

Prasad, S. and B.B. Aggarwal. "Turmeric, the golden spice," in I.F.F. Benzie et S. Wachtel-Galor, (dir.), *Herbal Medicine: Biomolecular and Clinical Aspects, 2nd edition*, Boca Raton (FL), CRC Press, 2011.

Lampe, J.W. "Spicing up a vegetarian diet: chemopreventive effects of phytochemicals," *Am J Clin Nutr* 2003; 78: 579S-583S.

Aggarwal, B.B. et al. "Curcumin-free turmeric exhibits anti-inflammatory and anticancer activities: identification of novel components of turmeric," *Mol Nutr Food Res* 2013; 57: 1529-42.

Gupta, S.C. et al. "Curcumin, a component of turmeric: from farm to pharmacy," *2013 BioFactors* 2013; 39: 2-13.

Bayet-Robert, M. et al. "Phase I dose escalation trial of docetaxel plus curcumin in patients with advanced and metastatic breast cancer," *Cancer Biol Ther* 2010; 9: 8-14.

Vankar, P.S. "Effectiveness of antioxidant properties of fresh and dry rhizomes of *Curcuma longa* (Long and Short Varieties) with dry turmeric spice," *Int J Food Eng* 1998; 4: 1-8.

Singh, G. et al. "Comparative study of chemical composition and antioxidant activity of fresh and dry rhizomes of turmeric (*Curcuma longa Linn.*)," *Food Chem Toxicol* 2010; 48: 1026-31.

Tayyem, R.F. et al. "Curcumin content of turmeric and curry powders," *Nutr Cancer* 2006; 55: 126-131.

Hoehle, S.I. et al. "Glucuronidation of curcuminoids by human microsomal and recombinant human UDP-glucuronosyltransferases," *Mol Nutr Food Res* 2007; 51: 932-8.

Shoba, G. et al. "Influence of piperine on the pharmacokinetics of curcumin in animals and human volunteers," *Planta Med* 1998; 64: 353-6.

Sehgal, A. et al. "Combined effects of curcumin and piperine in ameliorating benzo(a)pyrene induced DNA damage," *Food Chem Toxicol* 2011; 49: 3002-6.

Kakarala, M. et al. "Targeting breast stem cells with the cancer preventive compounds curcumin and piperine," *Breast Cancer Res Treat* 2010; 122: 777-85.

Dudhatra, G.B. et al. "A comprehensive review on pharmacotherapeutics of herbal bioenhancers," *Scientific World J* 2012; 2012: 637953.

Lamy, S. et al. "Diet-derived polyphenols inhibit angiogenesis by modulating the interleukin-6/STAT3 pathway," *Exp Cell Res* 2012; 318: 1586-96.

Lu, J. et al. "Novel angiogenesis inhibitory activity in cinnamon extract blocks VEGFR2 kinase and downstream signaling," *Carcinogenesis* 2010; 31: 481-8.

Surh, Y. "Molecular mechanisms of chemopreventive effects of selected dietary and medicinal phenolic substances," *Mutat Res* 1999; 428: 305-27.

Westerterp-Plantenga, M. et al. "Metabolic effects of spices, teas, and caffeine," *Physiol Behav* 2006; 89: 85-91.

Ludy, M.J. et al. "The effects of capsaicin and capsiate on energy balance: critical review and meta-analyses of studies in humans," *Chem Senses* 2012; 37: 103-121.

Chapter 9

Lanoë, C. "La céruse dans la fabrication des cosmétiques sous l'Ancien Régime (xvie-xviiie siècles)," *Techniques et Culture* 2002; 38, mis en ligne le 11 juillet 2006, consulté le 4 février 2014 (http://tc.revues.org/224).

www.liberation.fr/societe/2010/07/03/riviera-an-1_663489

http://jcdurbant.wordpress.com/2008/08/27/histoire-culturelle-linvention-du-bronzage-how-the-french-became-the-world's-tanning-masters/

Turck, L. *La vieillesse considérée comme maladie et les moyens de la combattre*, Paris, Victor Masson et fils, 1869.

Hirota, T. et al. "Identification of small molecule activators of cryptochrome," *Science* 2012; 337: 1094-1097.

Noonan, F.P. et al. "Melanoma induction by ultraviolet A but not ultraviolet B radiation requires melanin pigment," *Nat Commun* 2012; 3: 884.

Petersen, B. et al. "A sun holiday is a sunburn holiday," *Photodermatol Photoimmunol Photomed* 2013; 29: 221-4.

Bernard, J.J. et al. "Ultraviolet radiation damages self noncoding RNA and is detected by TLR3," *Nature Medicine* 2012; 18: 1286-1290.

Beleza, S. et al. "The timing of pigmentation lightening in Europeans," *Mol Biol Evol* 2013; 30: 24-35.

Halder, R.M. and S. Bridgeman-Shah. "Skin cancer in African Americans," *Cancer* 1995; 75 (Suppl. 2): 667-673.

Takeuchi, S. et al. "Melanin acts as a potent UVB photosensitizer to cause an atypical mode of cell death in murine skin," *Proc Natl Acad Sci USA* 2004; 101: 15076-81.

Mitra, D. et al. "An ultraviolet-radiation-independent pathway to melanoma carcinogenesis in the red hair/fair skin background," *Nature* 2012; 491: 449-543.

Fitzpatrick's Dermatology in General Medicine, Fifth Edition, New York, McGraw-Hill, 1999.

Cui, R. et al. "Central role of p53 in the suntan response and pathologic hyperpigmentation," *Cell* 2007; 128: 853-64.

Brash, D.E. "Roles of the transcription factor p53 in keratinocyte carcinomas," *Br J Dermatol* 2006; 154 Suppl 1: 8-10.

Oren, M. et J. Bartek. " The sunny side of p53," *Cell* 2007; 128: 826-8.

Miyamura, Y. et al. "The deceptive nature of UVA tanning versus the modest protective effects of UVB tanning on human skin," *Pigment Cell Melanoma Res* 2011; 24: 136-47.

www.planetesante.ch/Mag-sante/Cancer/Etre-bronze-ne-protege-pas-contre-le-cancer-de-la-peau

Mitchell, D. "Melanoma back in the UVA spotlight," *Pigment Cell Melanoma Res* 2013; 25: 540-541.

Zhang, M. "Use of tanning beds and incidence of skin cancer," *J Clin Oncol* 2012; 30: 1588-1593.

Noonan, F.P. et al. "Melanoma induction by ultraviolet A but not ultraviolet B radiation requires melanin pigment," *Nat Commun* 2012; 3: 884.

Elwood, J.M. and J. Jopson. "Melanoma and sun exposure: an overview of published studies," *Int J Cancer* 1997; 73: 198-203.

International Agency for Research on Cancer. "Solar and ultraviolet radiation," *IARC Monographs on the Evaluation of Carcinogenic Risks to Humans*, volume 55, Lyon, IARC Press, 1992.

Gandini, S. et al. "Meta-analysis of risk factors for cutaneous melanoma: 2. Sun exposure," *Eur Cancer* 2005; 41: 45-60.

Whiteman, D.C. et al. "Childhood sun exposure as a risk factor for melanoma: a systematic review of epidemiologic studies," *Cancer Causes Control* 2001; 12: 69-82.

D'Orazio, J.A. et al. "Melanoma: Epidemiology, Genetics and Risk Factors," in Lester M. Davids (dir.), *Recent Advances in the Biology, Therapy and Management of Melanoma*, Rijeka (Croatie), InTech, 2013 (http://dx.doi.org/10.5772/46052).

Parkin, D.M. et al. "Estimating the world cancer burden: Globocan 2000," *Int J Cancer* 2001; 94: 153-156.

www.medscape.com/viewarticle/470300_2

Moan, J. and A. Dahlback. "Predictions of health consequences of a changing UV-fluence," in L. Dubertret, R. Santus et P. Morliere (dir.), *Ozone, sun, cancer*, Paris, Inserm, 1995: 87-100.

Demers, A.A. et al. "Trends of nonmelanoma skin cancer from 1960 through 2000 in a Canadian population," *J Am Acad Derm* 2005; 53: 320-328.

www.dermatology.ca/fr/peau-cheveux-ongles/la-peau/cancer-de-la-peau/le-melanome-malin/

De Vries, E. et al. "Changing epidemiology of malignant cutaneous melanoma in Europe 1953-1997: rising trends in incidence and mortality but recent stabilizations in western Europe and decreases in Scandinavia," *Int J Cancer* 2003; 107: 19-26.

Autier, P. et al. "Sunscreen use and duration of sun exposure: A double blind randomized trial," *J Natl Cancer Inst* 1999; 15: 1304-1309.

Autier, P. et al. "Is sunscreen use for melanoma prevention valid for all sun exposure circumstances?," *J Clin Oncol* 2011; 29: e425-6.

International Agency for Research on Cancer, *IARC Handbooks of Cancer Prevention*, volume 5, Sunscreens, Lyon, IARC Press, 2001.

Green, A., G. Williams, R. Neale et al. "Daily sunscreen application and betacarotene supplementation in prevention of basal-cell and squamous-cell carcinomas of the skin: a randomised controlled trial," *Lancet* 1999; 354: 723-729.

Green, A.C., et al. "Reduced melanoma after regular sunscreen use: randomized control trial follow-up," *J Clin Oncol* 2011; 29: 257-263.

Williams, H. and A. Pembroke. "Sniffer dogs in the melanoma clinic?," *Lancet* 1989; 1: 734.

Ehmann, R. et al. "Canine scent detection in the diagnosis of lung cancer: Revisiting a puzzling phenomenon," *Eur Respir J* 2012; 39: 669-76.

Sonoda, H. et al. "Colorectal cancer screening with odour material by canine scent detection," *Gut* 2011; 60: 814-819.

Chapter 10

Parkin, D.M. "The global health burden of infection-associated cancers in the year 2002," *Int J Cancer* 2006; 118: 3030-3044.

www.cancer.org/cancer/cancercauses/othercarcinogens/infectiousagents/infectiousagentsandcancer/infectious-agents-and-cancer-viruses

Bosch, F.X. et al. "Comprehensive control of human papillomavirus infections and related diseases," *Vaccine* 2013; 31 Suppl 8: I1-31.

D'Souza, G. et al. "Case-control study of human papillomavirus and oropharyngeal cancer," *N Engl J Med* 2007; 356: 1944-56.

Chaturvedi, A.K. et al. "Human papillomavirus and rising oropharyngeal cancer incidence in the United States," *J Clin Oncol* 2011; 29: 4294-301.

Gillison, M.L. et al. "Prevalence of oral HPV infection in the United States, 2009-2010," *JAMA* 2012; 307: 693-703.

Herrero, R. et al. "Reduced prevalence of oral human papillomavirus (HPV) 4 years after bivalent HPV vaccination in a randomized clinical trial in Costa Rica," *PLoS One* 2013; 8: e68329.

www.philalethe.net/post/2006/03/03/245-a-quoi-bon-dormir

Xie, L. et al. "Sleep drives metabolite clearance from the adult brain," *Science* 2013; 342: 373-377.

Cohen, S. et al. "Sleep habits and susceptibility to the common cold," *Arch Intern Med* 2009; 169: 62-7.

Cappuccio, F.P. et al. "Sleep duration and all-cause mortality: a systematic review and meta-analysis of prospective studies," *Sleep* 2010; 33: 585-92.

Von Ruesten, A. et al. "Association of Sleep Duration with Chronic Diseases in the European Prospective Investigation into Cancer and Nutrition (EPIC) - Potsdam Study," *PLoS One* 2012; 7: e30972.

Lehrer, S. et al. "Obesity and deranged sleep are independently associated with increased cancer mortality in 50 US states and the District of Columbia," *Sleep Breath* 2013; 17: 1117-8.

Aggarwal, S. et al. "Associations Between Sleep Duration and Prevalence of Cardiovascular Events," *Clin Cardiol* 2013 [Epub avant publication].

Eguchi, K. et al. "Short sleep duration as an independent predictor of cardiovascular events in Japanese patients with hypertension," *Arch Intern Med* 2008; 168: 2225-2231.

Ayas, N.T. et al. "A prospective study of self-reported sleep duration and incident diabetes in women," *Diabetes Care* 2003; 26(2): 380-4.

Patel, S.R. "Reduced sleep as an obesity risk factor," *Obes Rev* 2009; 10 Suppl 2: 61-8.

Xiao, Q. et al. "A large prospective investigation of sleep duration, weight change, and obesity in the NIH-AARP Diet and Health Study cohort," *Am J Epidemiol* 2013; 178: 1600-10.

Hu, L.Y. et al. "The risk of cancer among patients with sleep disturbance: a nationwide retrospective study in Taiwan," *Ann Epidemiol* 2013; 23: 757-61.

Thompson, C.L. et al. "Short duration of sleep increases risk of colorectal adenoma," *Cancer* 2011; 117: 841-847.

Sigurdardottir, L.G. et al. "Sleep disruption among older men and risk of prostate cancer," *Cancer Epidemiol Biomarkers Prev* 2013; 22: 872-9.

Luo, J. et al. "Sleep disturbance and incidence of thyroid cancer in postmenopausal women the Women's Health Initiative," *Am J Epidemiol* 2013; 177: 42-9.

Vogtmann, E. et al. "Association between sleep and breast cancer incidence among postmenopausal women in the women's health initiative," *Sleep* 2013; 36: 1437-44.

Qin, Y. et al. "Sleep duration and breast cancer risk: a meta-analysis of observational studies," *Int J Cancer* 2014; 134: 1166-73.

Parent, M.-É. et al. "Night work and the risk of cancer among men," *Am. J. Epidemiol.* 2012; 176:751-9.

www.who.int/mediacentre/news/releases/2014/air-pollution/en/

Patel, S.R. et al. "A prospective study of sleep duration and mortality risk in women," *Sleep* 2004; 27: 440-4.

Zhang, X. et al. "Associations of self-reported sleep duration and snoring with colorectal cancer risk in men and women," *Sleep* 2013; 36: 681-8.

Leproult, R. and E. Van Cauter. "Role of sleep and sleep loss in hormonal release and metabolism," *Endocr Dev* 2010; 17: 11-21.

Nieto, F.J. et al. "Sleep-disordered breathing and cancer mortality: results from the Wisconsin sleep cohort study," *Am J Respir Crit Care Med* 2012; 186: 190-4.

Campos-Rodriguez, F. et al. "Association between obstructive sleep apnea and cancer incidence in a large multicenter Spanish cohort," *Am J Respir Crit Care Med* 2013; 187: 99-105.

Hakim, F. et al. "Fragmented sleep accelerates tumor growth and progression through recruitment of tumor-associated macrophages and TLR4 signaling," *Cancer Res* 2014 [Epub avant publication].

Luan, N.N. et al. "Breastfeeding and ovarian cancer risk: a meta-analysis of epidemiologic studies," *Am J Clin Nutr* 2013; 98: 1020-31.

www.nytimes.com/2013/12/02/opinion/bad-eating-habits-start-in-the-womb.html?_r=0

Vogt, M.C. et al. "Neonatal insulin action impairs hypothalamic neurocircuit formation in response to maternal high-fat feeding," *Cell* 2014; 156: 495-509.

Jadoulle, V. et al. "Le cancer, défaite du psychisme?," *Bull Cancer* 2004; 91: 249-56.

Nakaya, N. et al. "Personality traits and cancer risk and survival based on Finnish and Swedish registry data," *Am J Epidemiol* 2010; 172(4): 377-385.

Hansen, P.E. et al. "Personality traits, health behavior, and risk for cancer: a prospective study of Swedish twin court," *Cancer* 2005; 103: 1082-91.

Olsen, J.H. et al. "Cancer in the parents of children with cancer," *N Engl J Med* 1995; 333: 1594-1599.

Lambe, M. et al. "Maternal breast cancer risk after the death of a child," *Int J Cancer* 2004; 110: 763-6.

Sagi-Schwartz, A. et al. "Against all odds: genocidal trauma is associated with longer life-expectancy of the survivors," *PLoS One* 2013; 8: e69179.

Lemogne, C. et al. "Depression and the risk of cancer: A 15-year follow-up study of the GAZEL cohort," *Am J Epidemiol* 2013; 178: 1712-20.

Heikkilä, K. et al. "Work stress and risk of cancer: Meta-analysis of 5700 incident cancer events in 116,000 European men and women," *BMJ* 2013; 346: f165.

Nielsen, N.R. and M. Grønbaek. "Stress and cancer: a systematic update on the current knowledge," *Nat Clin Pract Oncol* 2006; 3: 612-20.

Savard, J. et al. "Natural course of insomnia comorbid with cancer: an 18-month longitudinal study," *J Clin Oncol* 2011; 29: 3580-6.

Irwin, M.R. et al. "Sleep disturbance, inflammation and depression risk in cancer survivors," *Brain Behav Immun* 2013; 30 Suppl: S58-67.

Lutgendorf, S.K. et al. "Host factors and cancer progression: biobehavioral signaling pathways and interventions," *J Clin Oncol* 2010; 28: 4094-9.

Mustian, K.M. et al. "Multicenter, randomized controlled trial of yoga for sleep quality among cancer survivors," *J Clin Oncol* 2013; 31: 3233-41.

Espie, C.A. et al. "Randomized controlled clinical effectiveness trial of cognitive behavior therapy compared with treatment as usual for persistent insomnia in patients with cancer," *J Clin Oncol* 2008; 26: 4651-4658.

Tirmarche, M. et al. "Lung Cancer Risk Associated with Low Chronic Radon Exposure: Results from the French Uranium Miners Cohort and the European Project" (www.irsn.fr/FR/Larecherche/publications-documentation/Publications_documentation/BDD_publi/DRPH/LEADS/Documents/IRPA10-P2A-56.pdf)

Auvinen, A. and G. Pershagen. "Indoor radon and deaths from lung cancer," *BMJ* 2009; 330: a3128.

Commission canadienne de sûreté nucléaire. "Le radon et la santé," Ministère de Transaux publics et Services gouvernementaux Canada, 2012.

Redberg, R.F. and R. Smith-Bindmanjan. "We Are Giving Ourselves Cancer," *The New York Times*, January 30, 2014.

Gray, A. et al. "Lung cancer deaths from indoor radon and the cost effectiveness and potential of policies to reduce them," *BMJ* 2009; 338: a3110.

International Agency for Research on Cancer. "Outdoor air pollution," *IARC Monographs on the Evaluation of Carcinogenic Risks to Humans*, volume 109, IARC [à paraître].

Lim, S.S. et al. "A comparative risk assessment of burden of disease and injury attributable to 67 risk factors and risk factor clusters in 21 regions, 1990-2010: a systematic analysis for the Global Burden of Disease Study 2010," *Lancet* 2012; 380: 2224-60.

www.epa.gov/airtrends/aqtrends.html

Diamanti-Kandarakis, E. et al. "Endocrine-disrupting chemicals: an Endocrine Society scientific statement," *Endocr Rev* 2009; 30:293-342.

Soto, A.M. and C. Sonnenschein. "Environmental causes of cancer: endocrine disruptors as carcinogens," *Nat Rev Endocrinol* 2010; 6:363-70.

Lamb, J.C. et al. "Critical comments on the WHO-UNEP State of the Science of Endocrine Disrupting Chemicals – 2012," *Regul Toxicol Pharmacol* 2014; 69: 22-40.

Brophy, J.T. et al. "Breast cancer risk in relation to occupations with exposure to carcinogens and endocrine disruptors: a Canadian case-control study," *Environ Health* 2012; 11: 87.

Rudel, R.A. et al. "New exposure biomarkers as tools for breast cancer epidemiology, biomonitoring, and prevention: a systematic approach based on animal evidence," *Environ Health Perspect* 2014 May 12. [Epub avant publication]

Mirick, D.K. et al. "Antiperspirant use and the risk of breast cancer," *J Natl Cancer Inst* 2002; 94: 1578-80.

Turati, F. et al. "Personal hair dye use and bladder cancer: a meta-analysis," *Ann Epidemiol* 2014; 24: 151-9.

Lim, U. et al. "Consumption of aspartame-containing beverages and incidence of hematopoietic and brain malignancies," *Cancer Epidemiol Biomarkers Prev* 2006; 15: 1654-1659.

Endo, M. et al. "Potential applications of carbon nanotubes," *Carbon Nanotubes* 2008; 11: 13-61.

Sargent, L.M. et al. "Promotion of lung adenocarcinoma following inhalation exposure to multi-walled carbon nanotubes," *Part Fibre Toxicol* 2014; 11: 3.

Stewart, B.W. and C.P. Wild, dir. *World Cancer Report 2014*, IARC, OMS, 2014.

Ekenga, C.C. et al. "Breast cancer risk after occupational solvent exposure: the influence of timing and setting," *Cancer Res* 2014; 74: 3076-3083.

Egner, P. A et al. "Rapid and sustainable detoxication of airborne pollutants by broccoli sprout beverage: results of a randomized clinical trial in China," *Cancer Prev Res* 2014 June 9. pii:canprevres.0103.2014 [Epub avant publication]

Chapter 11

Macpherson, H. et al. "Multivitamin-multimineral supplementation and mortality: a meta-analysis of randomized controlled trials," *Am J Clin Nutr* 2013; 97: 437-44.

Bjelakovic, G. et al. "Antioxidant supplements and mortality," *Curr Opin Clin Nutr Metab Care* 2013 Nov 14.

Ristow, M. and S. Schmeisser. "Extending life span by increasing oxidative stress," *Free Radic Biol Med* 2011; 51: 327-36.

Albanes, D. et al. "Alpha-Tocopherol and beta-carotene supplements and lung cancer incidence in the alpha-tocopherol, beta-carotene cancer prevention study: effects of base-line characteristics and study compliance," *J Natl Cancer Inst* 1996; 88: 1560-70.

The Alpha-Tocopherol, Beta Carotene Cancer Prevention Study Group. "The effect of vitamin E and beta carotene on the incidence of lung cancer and other cancers in male smokers," *N Engl J Med* 1994; 330: 1029-35.

Omenn, G.S. et al. "Risk factors for lung cancer and for intervention effects in CARET, the Beta-Carotene and Retinol Efficacy Trial," *J Natl Cancer Inst* 1996; 88: 1550-9.

Bjelakovic, G. et al. "Antioxidant supplements for preventing gastrointestinal cancers," *Cochrane Database Syst Rev* 2008; CD004183.

Miller, E.R. "Meta-analysis: high-dosage vitamin E supplementation may increase all-cause mortality," *Ann Intern Med* 2005; 142: 37-46.

Lonn, E. et al. "Effects of long-term vitamin E supplementation on cardiovascular events and cancer: a randomized controlled trial," *JAMA* 2005; 293: 1338-47.

Lawson, K.A. et al. "Multivitamin use and risk of prostate cancer in the National Institutes of Health-AARP Diet and Health Study," *J Natl Cancer Inst* 2007; 99: 754-64.

Mursu, J. et al. "Dietary supplements and mortality rate in older women: the Iowa Women's Health Study," *Arch Intern Med* 2011; 171: 1625-33.

Klein, E.A. et al. "Vitamin E and the risk of prostate cancer: the Selenium and Vitamin E Cancer Prevention Trial (SELECT)," *JAMA* 2011; 306: 1549-56.

Xu, H. et al. "An international trial of antioxidants in the prevention of preeclampsia (INTAPP)," *Am J Obstet Gynecol* 2010; 202: 239.

Watson, J. "Oxidants, antioxidants and the current incurability of metastatic cancers," *Open Biol* 2013; 3: 120144.

Bairati, I. et al. "Randomized trial of antioxidant vitamins to prevent acute adverse effects of radiation therapy in head and neck cancer patients," *J Clin Oncol* 2005; 23: 5805-13.

Clarke, J.D. et al. "Comparison of isothiocyanate metabolite levels and histone deacetylase activity in human subjects consuming broccoli sprouts or broccoli supplement," *J Agric Food Chem* 2011; 59: 10955-63.

Hoshi, T. et al. "Omega-3 fatty acids lower blood pressure by directly activating large-conductance Ca2+-dependent K+ channels," *Proc Natl Acad Sci USA* 2013; 110: 4816-21.

Garland, C.F. and F.C. Garland. "Do sunlight and vitamin D reduce the likelihood of colon cancer?," *Int J Epidemiol* 1980; 9: 227-31.

Van der Rhee, H. et al. "Is prevention of cancer by sun exposure more than just the effect of vitamin D? A systematic review of epidemiological studies," *Eur J Cancer* 2013; 49: 1422-36.

Lappe, J.M. et al. "Vitamin D and calcium supplementation reduces cancer risk: results of a randomized trial," *Am J Clin Nutr* 2007; 85: 1586-1591.

Cheng, T.Y. et al. "Vitamin D intake and lung cancer risk in the Women's Health Initiative," *Am J Clin Nutr* 2013; 98: 1002-11.

Schöttker, B. et al. "Strong associations of 25-hydroxyvitamin D concentrations with all-cause, cardiovascular, cancer, and respiratory disease mortality in a large cohort study," *Am J Clin Nutr* 2013; 97: 782-93.

Goodwin, P.J. et al. "Prognostic effects of 25-hydroxyvitamin D levels in early breast cancer," *J Clin Oncol* 2009; 27: 3757-63.

Vrieling, A. et al. "Circulating 25-hydroxyvitamin D and postmenopausal breast cancer survival: influence of tumor characteristics and lifestyle factors?," *Int J Cancer* 2013 Nov 22.

Moan, J. et al. "Seasonal variations of cancer incidence and prognosis," *Dermatoendocrinol* 2010; 2: 55-7.

Zhou, W. et al. "Vitamin D is associated with overall survival in early stage non-small cell lung cancer patients," *Cancer Epidemiol Biomarkers Prev* 2005; 14: 2303-9.

Giovannucci, E. et al. "Prospective study of predictors of vitamin D status and cancer incidence and mortality in men," *J Natl Cancer Inst* 2006; 98: 451-459.

Vieth, R. "Vitamin D supplementation, 25-hydroxyvitamin D concentrations, and safety," *Am J Clin Nutr* 1999; 69: 842-856.

Houghton, L.A. and R. Vieth. "The case against ergocalciferol (vitamin D2) as a vitamin supplement," *Am J Clin Nutr* 2006; 84: 694-7.

Feldman, D. et al. "The role of Vitamin D in reducing cancer risk and progression," *Nat Rev Cancer* 2014; 14: 342-57.

Chapter 12

American Cancer Society. *Cancer Facts & Figures 2011* (www.cancer.org/acs/groups/content/@epidemiologysurveilance/documents/document/acspc-029771.pdf).

Williams, K. et al. "Is a cancer diagnosis a trigger for health behaviour change? Findings from a prospective, population-based study," *Br J Cancer* 2013; 108: 2407-12.

Skeie, G. et al. "Dietary change among breast and colorectal cancer survivors and cancer-free women in the Norwegian Women and Cancer cohort study," *Cancer Causes Control* 2009; 20: 1955-66.

Demark-Wahnefried, W. et al. "Riding the crest of the teachable moment: promoting long-term health after the diagnosis of cancer," *J Clin Oncol* 2005; 23: 5814-5830.

Tao, L. et al. "Impact of postdiagnosis smoking on long-term survival of cancer patients: the Shanghai cohort study," *Cancer Epidemiol Biomarkers Prev* 2013; 22: 2404-11.

Munro, A.J. et al. "Smoking compromises cause-specific survival in patients with operable colorectal cancer," *Clin Oncol* 2006; 18: 436-40.

Ehlers, S.L. et al. "The impact of smoking on outcomes among patients undergoing hematopoietic SCT for the treatment of acute leukemia," *Bone Marrow Transplant* 2011; 46: 285-90.

Braithwaite, D. et al. "Smoking and survival after breast cancer diagnosis: a prospective observational study and systematic review," *Breast Cancer Res Treat* 2012; 136: 521-33.

Protani, M. et al. "Effect of obesity on survival of women with breast cancer: Systematic review and meta-analysis," *Breast Cancer Res Treat* 2010; 123: 627-35.

Abrahamson, P.E. et al. "General and abdominal obesity and survival among young women with breast cancer," *Cancer Epidemiol Biomarkers Prev* 2006; 15: 1871-7.

Parekh, N. et al. "Obesity in cancer survival," *Annu Rev Nutr* 2012; 32: 311-42.

Ma, J. et al. "Prediagnostic body-mass index, plasma C-peptide concentration, and prostate cancer-specific mortality in men with prostate cancer: a long-term survival analysis," *Lancet Oncol* 2008; 9: 1039-47.

Beasley, J.M. et al. "Post-diagnosis dietary factors and survival after invasive breast cancer," *Breast Cancer Res Treat* 2011; 128: 229-36.

Meyerhardt, J.A. et al. "Dietary glycemic load and cancer recurrence and survival in patients with stage III colon cancer: findings from CALGB 89803," *J Natl Cancer Inst* 2012; 104: 1702-11.

Meyerhardt, J.A. "We are what we eat, or are we?," *J Clin Oncol* 2013; 31: 2763-4.

McCullough, M.L. et al. "Association between red and processed meat intake and mortality among colorectal cancer survivors," *J Clin Oncol* 2013; 31: 2773-82.

Zhu, Y. et al. "Dietary patterns and colorectal cancer recurrence and survival: a cohort study," *BMJ Open* 2013; 3: pii: e002270.

Meyerhardt, J.A. et al. "Association of dietary patterns with cancer recurrence and survival in patients with stage III colon cancer," *JAMA* 2007; 298: 754-764.

Vrieling, A. et al. "Dietary patterns and survival in German postmenopausal breast cancer survivors," *Br J Cancer* 2013; 108: 188-92.

Kwan, M.L. et al. "Dietary patterns and breast cancer recurrence and survival among women with early-stage breast cancer," *J Clin Oncol* 2009; 27: 919-26.

Wayne, S.J. et al. "Changes in dietary intake after diagnosis of breast cancer," *J Am Diet Assoc* 2004; 104: 1561-1568.

Milliron, B.J. et al. "Usual dietary intake among female breast cancer survivors is not significantly different from women with no cancer history: results of the National Health and Nutrition Examination Survey, 2003-2006," *J Acad Nutr Diet* 2013; pii: S2212-2672(13)01339-7.

Guha, N. et al. "Soy isoflavones and risk of cancer recurrence in a cohort of breast cancer survivors: the Life After Cancer Epidemiology study," *Breast Cancer Res Treat* 2009; 118: 395-405.

Shu, X.O. et al. "Soy food intake and breast cancer survival," *JAMA* 2009; 302: 2437-2443.

Chi, F. et al. "Post-diagnosis soy food intake and breast cancer survival: a meta-analysis of cohort studies," *Asian Pac J Cancer Prev* 2013; 14: 2407-12.

Nechuta, S.J. et al. "Soy food intake after diagnosis of breast cancer and survival: an in-depth analysis of combined evidence from cohort studies of US and Chinese women," *Am J Clin Nutr* 2012; 96: 123-32.

Kang, X. et al. "Effect of soy isoflavones on breast cancer recurrence and death for patients receiving adjuvant endocrine therapy," *CMAJ* 2010; 182: 1857-62.

McCann, S.E. et al. "Dietary lignan intakes in relation to survival among women with breast cancer: The Western New York Exposures and Breast Cancer (WEB) Study," *Breast Cancer Res Treat* 2010; 122: 229-35.

Munday, R. et al. "Inhibition of urinary bladder carcinogenesis by broccoli sprouts," *Cancer Res* 2008; 68: 1593-600.

Tang, L. et al. "Intake of cruciferous vegetables modifies bladder cancer survival," *Cancer Epidemiol Biomarkers Prev* 2010; 19: 1806-11.

Thomson, C.A. et al. "Vegetable intake is associated with reduced breast cancer recurrence in tamoxifen users: a secondary analysis from the Women's Healthy Eating and Living Study," *Breast Cancer Res Treat* 2011; 125: 519-527.

Chan, J.M. et al. "Diet after diagnosis and the risk of prostate cancer progression, recurrence, and death (United States)," *Cancer Causes Control* 2006; 17(2): 199-208.

Ogunleye, A.A. et al. "Green tea consumption and breast cancer risk or recurrence: a meta-analysis," *Breast Cancer Res Treat* 2010; 119: 477-484.

Physical Activity Guidelines Advisory Committee report, 2008. "To the Secretary of Health and Human Services. Part A: executive summary," *Nutr Rev* 2008; 67(2): 114-120.

Schmitz, K.H. et al. "American College of Sports Medicine roundtable on exercise guidelines for cancer survivors," *Medicine and Science in Sports and Exercise* 2010; 42: 1409-1426.

Ballard-Barbash, R. et al. "Physical activity, biomarkers, and disease outcomes in cancer survivors: a systematic review," *J Natl Cancer Inst* 2012; 104: 815-40.

Irwin, M.L. et al. "Physical activity and survival in postmenopausal women with breast cancer: results from the women's health initiative," *Cancer Prev Res* 2011; 4: 522-529.

Friedenreich, C.M. et al. "Prospective cohort study of lifetime physical activity and breast cancer survival," *Int J Cancer* 2009; 124: 1954-62.

Holick, C.N. et al. "Physical activity and survival after diagnosis of invasive breast cancer," *Cancer Epidemiol Biomarkers Prev* 2008; 17: 379-86.

Irwin, M.L. et al. "Influence of pre- and postdiagnosis physical activity on mortality in breast cancer survivors: the health, eating, activity, and lifestyle study," *J Clin Oncol* 2008; 26: 3958-64.

Meyerhardt, J.A. et al. "Physical activity and male colorectal cancer survival," *Arch Intern Med* 2009; 169: 2102-8.

Meyerhardt, J.A. et al. "Physical activity and survival after colorectal cancer diagnosis," *J Clin Oncol* 2006; 24: 3527-34.

Kenfield, S.A. et al. "Physical activity and survival after prostate cancer diagnosis in the health professionals follow-up study," *J Clin Oncol* 2011; 29: 726-732.

Moorman, P.G. et al. "Recreational physical activity and ovarian cancer risk and survival," *Ann Epidemiol* 2011; 21: 178-187.

Ruden, E. et al. "Exercise behavior, functional capacity, and survival in adults with malignant recurrent glioma," *J Clin Oncol* 2011; 29: 2918-2923.

Barone, B.B. et al. "Long-term all-cause mortality in cancer patients with preexisting diabetes mellitus: a systematic review and meta-analysis," *JAMA* 2008; 300: 2754-64.

Reynolds, G. "Cancer Survivors Who Stay Active Live Longer," *The New York Times*, 16 mai 2012.

Giovannucci, E.L. "Physical activity as a standard cancer treatment," *J Natl Cancer Inst* 2012; 104: 797-9.

Reding, K.W. et al. "Effect of prediagnostic alcohol consumption on survival after breast cancer in young women," *Cancer Epidemiol Biomarkers Prev* 2008; 17: 1988-96.

Barnett, G.C. et al. "Risk factors for the incidence of breast cancer: do they affect survival from the disease?," *J Clin Oncol* 2008; 26: 3310-6.

Flatt, S.W. et al. "Low to moderate alcohol intake is not associated with increased mortality after breast cancer," *Cancer Epidemiol Biomarkers Prev* 2010; 19: 681-8.

Kwan, M.L. et al. "Postdiagnosis alcohol consumption and breast cancer prognosis in the after breast cancer pooling project," *Cancer Epidemiol Biomarkers Prev* 2013; 22: 32-41.

Kwan, M.L. et al. "Alcohol consumption and breast cancer recurrence and survival among women with early-stage breast cancer: The Life After Cancer Epidemiology (LACE) Study," *J Clin Oncol* 2010; 28: 4410-4416.

Harris, H.R. et al. "Alcohol intake and mortality among women with invasive breast cancer," *Br J Cancer* 2012; 106: 592-5.

Holmes, M.D. "Challenge of balancing alcohol intake," *J Clin Oncol* 2010; 28: 4403-4.

Zell, J.A. et al. "Differential effects of wine consumption on colorectal cancer outcomes based on family history of the disease," *Nutr Cancer* 2007; 59: 36-45.

Velicer, C.M. and C.M. Ulrich. "Vitamin and mineral supplement use among US adults after cancer diagnosis: a systematic review," *J Clin Oncol* 2008; 26: 665-73.

Miller, P. et al. "Dietary supplement use among elderly, long-term cancer survivors," *J Cancer Surviv* 2008; 2: 138-48.

Rock, C.L. et al. "Nutrition and physical activity guidelines for cancer survivors," *CA Cancer J Clin* 2012; 62: 243-74.

Davies, A.A. et al. "Nutritional interventions and outcome in patients with cancer or preinvasive lesions: systematic review," *J Natl Cancer Inst* 2006; 98: 961-73.

Kwan, M.L. et al. "Multivitamin use and breast cancer outcomes in women with early-stage breast cancer: The Life After Cancer Epidemiology study," *Breast Cancer Res Treat* 2011; 130: 195-205.

Harris, H.R. et al. "Vitamin C intake and breast cancer mortality in a cohort of Swedish women," *Br J Cancer* 2013; 109: 257-64.

Poole, E.M. et al. "Postdiagnosis supplement use and breast cancer prognosis in the After Breast Cancer Pooling Project," *Breast Cancer Res Treat* 2013; 139: 529-37.

Ng, K. et al. "Multivitamin use is not associated with cancer recurrence or survival in patients with stage III colon cancer: findings from CALGB 89803," *J Clin Oncol* 2010; 28: 4354-63.

Figueiredo, J.C. et al. "Folic acid and prevention of colorectal adenomas: a combined analysis of randomized clinical trials," *Int J Cancer* 2011; 129: 192-203.

Greenlee, H. et al. "Antioxidant supplement use after breast cancer diagnosis and mortality in the Life After Cancer Epidemiology (LACE) cohort," *Cancer* 2012; 118: 2048-58.

Baron, J.A. et al. "Neoplastic and antineoplastic effects of beta-carotene on colorectal adenoma recurrence: results of a randomized trial," *J Natl Cancer Inst* 2003; 95: 717-722.

Bairati, I. et al. "Antioxidant vitamins supplementation and mortality: a randomized trial in head and neck cancer patients," *Int J Cancer* 2006; 119: 2221-2224.

IMAGE CREDITS

Getty Images

C1: Jonya/E+; C4-A: David Job/Stockbyte; C4-B: Digital Vision; C4-C: Bruce Yuanyue Bi/Lonely Planet Images; C4-D: Brand X Pictures; 2: Buyenlarge/Time Life Pictures; 6: Tim MacPherson/Riser; 9: Ineke Kamps/Moment; 10: Rubberball; 12: Leon Neal/AFP; 13: David Mack/Science Photo Library; 15: Tim Flach/Stone; 17: Baris Simsek/E+; 18: Peter Dazeley/Photographer's Choice; 21: Benoit Paillé/Moment Select; 22: Camazine Scott/Photo Researchers; 24: sozaijiten/Datacraft; 25: Frans Lanting/Mint Images; 27: Adrianna Williams/Stone; 28: Jeff J Mitchell News; 29: Dean Mitchell/E+; 30: Purestock; 31: coloroftime/E+; 34: Digital Vision; 35: OJO Images; 36: David Job/Stockbyte; 39: Popperfoto; 40: Ray Pfortner/Photolibrary; 41: Narvikk/E+; 43: Charlie Abad/Photononstop; 44: Tim Hawley/Photographer's Choice; 46: Culture Club/Hulton Archive; 47: Hulton Archive; 48: Media for Medical/Universal Images Group; 49: Goh Chai Hin/AFP; 50-A: M Daugherty John/Photo Researchers; 50-B: Arthur Glauberman/Photo Researchers; 52: SMC Images/Photodisc; 53: Fuse; 54: Nemanja Glumac/Vetta; 55: Art Glazer/Photodisc; 56: Media for Medical/Universal Images Group; 58: Joan Vicent Cantó Roig/Vetta; 60: Todd Wright/Blend Images; 62: Godong/Universal Images Group; 65: Jeff haynes/AFP; 67: Peter Dazeley/Photographer's Choice; 69: Steve Gschmeissner/Science Photo Library; 71: Marcela Barsse/E+; 72: Steven Puetzer/Photographer's Choice RF; 74: Scott Olson News; 75: Pornchai/AFP; 76: Kelly Cline/E+; 78: Dan McCoy–Rainbow/Science Faction; 79: Age fotostock; 81: Daniel Mihailescu/AFP; 82: Michele Pauty/ASABlanca; 83: Maria Toutoudaki/Photodisc; 85: Nathan Jones/Vetta; 87: Bloomberg; 88: Lorenzo Dominguez/Moment; 93: Smneedham/Photolibrary; 94: Tony C French/Digital Vision; 95: Christopher Pillitz/The Image Bank; 98: Sandeep Subba/Vetta; 100: Yagi Studio/Digital Vision; 102: DEA/G. Dagli Orti/De Agostini Picture Library; 106: John Block/Blend Images; 108: Aleaimage/E+; 111: Ermin Gutenberger/E+; 113: Brian Macdonald/Digital Vision; 115: Chris Stein/Stockbyte; 116: Sonja Dahlgren/Maskot; 119: Jessica Peterson; 120: Robert Churchill/Vetta; 121: BJI/Blue Jean Images; 123-A: John Block/Blend Images/Getty Images; 124: rzdeb/E+; 128: White Rock; 130: Ryan Heffernan/Aurora; 131: Tom Grill/Photographer's Choice RF; 132: Pawel Libera/Light Rocket; 135: Blend Images–KidStock/Brand X Pictures; 136: Anna Pekunova/Moment Open; 137: Robert Holmgren/The Image Bank; 138: Chris Cheadle/All Canada Photos; 139: Phillip Hayson/Photodisc; 140: Apostrophe Productions/Photlibrary; 141: JGI/Tom Grill/Blend Images; 144: Westend61/Brand X Pictures; 147: Foodcollection RF; 148: Tim Graham News; 149: Ghislain & Marie David de Lossy/The Image Bank; 152: Purestock; 153: Ollie Millington Entertainment; 155: Christopher Badzioch/E+; 156-A: Datacraft Co Ltd; 157: GSO Images/Photographer's Choice RF; 160: Ariel Skelley/Blend Images; 162: Mark Wragg/E+; 165: Dmytro Tokar/E+; 166: Jean-Luc Manaud/Gamma Rapho via Getty Images; 167: Ingram Publishing/Vetta; 168: MedicalRF.com; 169: Paul Bernhardt/Dorling Kindersley; 170: Neo Vision/amana images; 171: Steve Bronstein/The Image Bank; 172: Philip Wilkins/Photolibrary; 174: Maren Caruso/Digital Vision; 175: Jupiterimages/Photolibrary; 176: John Turner/The Image Bank; 177: Burwell and Burwell Photography/E+; 178: Alina Vincent Photography, LLC/E+; 180: Synergee/E+; 181: Floortje/E+; 182: DEA/G. Dagli Orti/De Agostini Picture Library.; 184: Steven Errico/Photographer's Choice RF; 185: TommL/Vetta; 186: loops7/E+; 189: NASA/Science Photo Library; 190: Bob Thomas/E+; 191: Philip Lee Harvey/Photonica World; 193: Daniel MacDonald/Moment; 194: George Rose Entertainment; 195: Kallista Images; 196: Bruce Yuanyue Bi/Lonely Planet Images; 198: CMSP; 198: Dr. Kenneth Greer/Visuals Unlimited; 198: Tom Myers/Photo Researchers; 199: E+; 200: NIBSC/Science Photo Library; 202B: Photo Researchers; 203: Science Picture Co/Collection Mix: Subjects; 205: Science Photo Library-Ian Hooton/Brand X Pictures; 206: ChinaFotoPress via Getty Images; 211: J. Chech/Science Foto; 214: Digital Vision; 215: peter zelei/Vetta; 216: knape/Vetta; 218: VikaValter/Vetta; 220: Bloomberg via Getty Images; 221: Danita Delimont/Gallo Images; 222: Ann Cutting/Photographer's Choice; 224: Westend61; 227: Martin Wimmer/E+; 228: Antonio M. Rosario/Photographer's Choice; 229: Yuji Sakai/Photodisc; 230: kristian sekulic/E+; 234: Coneyl Jay/Stone; 236: skynesher/Vetta; 238: Jessica Key/E+; 240: Hiroshi Watanabe/Stockbyte; 241: Assembly/Stone; 243: Michael Courtney/E+; 244: Hero Images; 247: Mary Gascho/Vetta; 248: Purestock

Michel Rouleau

14, 20, 26, 42, 57, 68, 142, 145, 151, 188

Shutterstock

19: oliveromg; 23: leolintang; 32A: Lasse Kristensen; 32B, 125, 209: Africa Studio; 32C: Volosina; 32D: NataliTerr; 32E: George Dolgikh; 33A: somchaij; 33B: Yalcin Sonat; 33C: Robert Kneschke; 33D: Vucicevic Milos; 33E: Lisa F. Young; 38: Sam Murray; 45: Michael-John Wolfe; 51: Alan Bailey; 53B: Aleksandrs Samuilovs; 61: Giuseppe_R; 63: kiboka; 64: wavebreakmedia; 66: aboikis; 84: Niloo; 89: Bangkokhappiness; 90A: Regele Ionescu; 90B, 90C: Sassan Lee-Kramer; 92A: Palo_ok; 92B: wasa_d; 96: branislavpudar; 97: Marafona; 99: Jacek Chabraszewski; 103: Bud Leigh-Humes; 104: Hong Vo; 105: szefei; 107: Tagstock1; 109: Sal Hadt; 110: WBB; 112: wavebreakmedia 114: Karen Faljyan; 118: Givaga; 122: Zb89V; 123: bonchan; 126: Angel Simon; 127: Yasonya; 133: ArtFamily; 134: ostill; 156: Pavel Isupov; 159: Vince Clements; 161: somchaij; 164: PanicAttack; 170: Elena Elisseeva; 173: Andrii Gorulko; 192: Bazán Nhey; 197: Alexander Raths; 198: Jame-Sally Picault; 202: Image Point Fr; 212: Tyler Olson; 222: Monticello; 225: Sally-Ann O'Hara; 231: Kellis; 232: JPC-Prod; 235, 237: Alexander Raths

INDEX